SELF-MASSAGE

About the Author

Jacqueline Young is a clinical psychologist and acupuncturist who lived for four and a half years in Japan studying and practising oriental medicine. She has also travelled widely in India and the Far East studying traditional health techniques. She is a visiting lecturer at the Centre for Complementary Health Studies, University of Exeter and the author of books and articles on natural medicine.

SELF-MASSAGE

A complete 15-minutes-a-day
massage system
for health and healing

JACQUELINE YOUNG

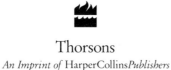

Thorsons
An Imprint of HarperCollins*Publishers*

Thorsons
An Imprint of HarperCollins*Publishers*
77-85 Fulham Palace Road
Hammersmith, London W6 8JB

Published by Thorsons 1992
10 9 8 7 6 5 4 3 2

A catalogue record for this book
is available from the British Library

ISBN 0 7225 2510 9

Printed in Great Britain by
Butler & Tanner, Frome, Somerset

Photographs by Peter Chadwick
Line illustrations by Andrea Darlow

For Sarah

Acknowledgements

With many thanks to my Japanese, Chinese and Tibetan teachers, and to my students in the East and West; to Caroline Faulkner and Nigel Dawes for their modelling; to Peter Chadwick and his assistant, Brenda Peringer, for the photography and all their good humour; to Tinks Reading, make-up artist; to Andrea Darlow for the illustrations; to John Hardaker for starting things at Thorsons and to Jane Graham-Maw, Rosamund Saunders and Zoë Maggs for seeing the project to completion; to Frances Kelly for her work as agent; to Gill Palmer and Chris McLaughlin for their typing; to Nic and Kirsten for their companionship, warmth and love; and to Nick, for keeping me happy when the going got tough!

Contents

INTRODUCTION

1 Why self-massage?

The art of massage has been with us since ancient times. It can be used for relaxation and pleasure, or therapeutically in the treatment of aches, pain and injuries.

In the Orient, self-massage techniques have traditionally been handed down in families, and sometimes even taught in schools, for the relief of tension and the promotion of health.

There are many techniques of massage, and some take several years and much practice to master. Yet each have simple movements which can easily be learnt and used to good effect on one's own body.

By learning how to massage yourself you can:

- build up good health and prevent disease
- aid relaxation
- promote healing of minor ailments and imbalances
- increase self-awareness

Anyone can learn self-massage and, with practice, you can vitalize the whole body in a 15 minute top-to-toe routine. Alternatively, just a few minutes can be spent massaging whichever part of the body requires attention:

for example, massaging the neck and shoulders to relieve a stiff neck or headache.

With this massage you will have a self-health system literally at your fingertips! It can be used anytime, anywhere, and no special equipment or oils are needed. It is not even necessary to remove clothing as the techniques are designed to be performed through light clothing as easily as on the skin itself.

Once you feel confident of the movements they can easily be adapted for use on others. So, by learning self-massage, friends and family can benefit too!

With self-massage, because you are working on yourself, you can practise whenever you have a free moment rather than having to find someone to practise on. This means that you can quickly build up confidence in your touch and develop mastery of the techniques.

With experience you will learn to detect subtle changes in the body which can be a valuable tool in monitoring your health and determining the body's needs. Regular practice will ensure relief from tiredness and tension and will leave you feeling vibrant and well.

2 The self-massage system

This simple self-massage system is based on a combination of Japanese and Chinese massage therapies, together with acupressure techniques. The system works not only on releasing muscular tension, but also on stimulating the energetic system of the body, known in acupuncture as the meridian system.

The meridians

According to oriental medical theory, a network of channels covers the entire body and links with each of the internal organs. These channels, or meridians, are located just below the surface of the skin. They are not visible to the naked eye but can be measured electrically. They are said to conduct a current through the body which is termed 'Qi' in Chinese and 'Ki' in Japanese, and is generally translated as 'vital energy'. The balanced supply of this vital energy throughout the body is said to be essential for health. There are twelve main meridians; they function in pairs and run on both sides of the body. There are also eight extraordinary meridians, two of which are important in the self-massage system.

The twelve main meridians
> Lung – Large Intestine
> Stomach – Spleen
> Heart – Small Intestine
> Urinary Bladder – Kidney
> Pericardium – Triple Heater
> Gall Bladder – Liver

Two extraordinary meridians
> Conception Vessel – Governor Vessel

Most of the meridians correspond to actual physical organs, but others relate to specific functions of the body. The Triple Heater meridian relates to circulation and the distribution of fluids around the body, as well as to the health of the sexual organs. The pericardium is a membrane around the heart and the Pericardium meridian relates to heart and circulatory function in the body. The Conception and Governor Vessel meridians serve to supply and unite the energy within the other twelve meridians.

Acupoints

Along each meridian line there are points known as acupoints. These can be stimulated in order to influence the flow of vital energy in the meridian. In this massage system, fingertip pressure on the acupoints is used to clear blockages and maintain a balanced flow of energy throughout the body. Acupoints on each of the twelve main meridians are massaged on both sides of the body.

Because each of the meridians are said to connect with the internal organs, massage of acupoints can affect seemingly unrelated parts of the body. For example, massaging the acupoint, Stomach 36 on the leg can affect the workings of the stomach.

The acupoints are named according to the meridian on which they lie, and are numbered according to where they are on that meridian line. The names and numbers enable you to cross-reference the acupoints with any other acupressure or acupuncture texts.

Techniques

The self-massage techniques have been chosen for their simplicity and effectiveness. Their combination is based on many years of clinical practice and sessions with students in both East and West. The massage techniques help to release tension and promote a sense of well-being, while the acupressure works directly on the meridian system and helps to balance the internal organs.

Self-massage

The self-massage system is very adaptable. It provides the basis for a unique daily health routine that can be completed in a short time. The movements can also easily be modified to suit individual preferences or needs. By being sensitive to exactly what your body needs, at any given time, you can get the best out of this system and learn to give of your best, too.

3 Preparation

No special preparation is necessary for self-massage, but it helps if you take a few deep breaths and have a good stretch before starting. Many of the movements can be performed whenever you have a few spare minutes. For example: sitting in a chair at home, at a desk in the office, while waiting for a bus, standing in a queue or when in bed. However, if you are at home and want to do the complete self-massage and give yourself a real treat, then the following will help you get the best out of the massage:

- *Allow enough free time to complete your massage.* You will need a minimum of 15 minutes to work through the whole body, but can make the massage last longer if you wish.
- *Choose a comfortable place.* Either indoors or outside, with comfortable light, temperature and ventilation, and away from loud noise or strong smells if possible.
- *Wear comfortable, loose clothing.* If you wish to change, then a loose tracksuit is ideal. If not, simply loosen any tight clothing and remove shoes, belts, watches and jewellery.

- *Find a comfortable surface.* Either on a carpet or mat, in a chair or on grass – whatever suits you.
- *Remember to breathe* freely and deeply throughout the self-massage, synchronizing the movements with the breath if you can.
- *Adopt a comfortable position* for each movement. You should always be comfortable and relaxed without any pain or strain.
- *Avoid interruptions.* Do the self-massage at a time when you won't be interrupted and can give yourself your whole attention and loving care.

It is also advisable:

- to allow an hour after meals before starting.
- to avoid practising when either very tired or very hungry. Take a rest or have a snack first.
- not to smoke or drink coffee, tea or alcohol directly before practice.

All the above will help you to establish a healthy and enjoyable routine and to maximize the benefits of the self-massage.

4 *The sequence*

To help your initial practice the self-massage techniques have been arranged in a sequence according to body part. This helps you to remember the massage movements and to make sure that no part of the body has been missed out.

However, this sequence is only a starting point. Once you become confident of the moves, and increase your sensitivity, you will be able to adapt the sequence to your own needs. You must decide the best way for you and be ready to change it as you yourself change.

In general the sequence moves from the top to the bottom of the body and from the inside to the outside. This is in order to balance energy within the body as a whole and to stimulate the flow of energy from the central organs through to the periphery. Many people today have a surplus of energy in the upper part of the body, through an excess of mental activity and stress, and a lack of energy in the lower body, often resulting from sedentary jobs. Typical symptoms of this energy imbalance are: headaches, eye problems and neck and shoulder stiffness, together with weakness in the legs, cold feet, digestive problems and low back pain.

By working from the top to the bottom of the body the surplus energy is drawn away from over-burdened areas and used to nourish areas with a weak supply. A marked improvement in many of the above symptoms can be obtained within a short time using self-massage.

The sequence is divided up according to five areas of the body:

1 Head and face
2 Neck, shoulders and arms
3 Chest and abdomen
4 Back
5 Legs and feet

There is also a brief warm-up section and additional sections on breathing techniques and finger exercises.

When you are first learning this system it is a good idea to spend a few days on each area exclusively, until you have mastered the sequence of moves. Once you are familiar with the massage for each area you can then start putting them together to massage your body as a whole.

Alternatively, you can add a new area of your body each time you practise. For example: learn the head and face massage one day; the next day perform the head and face massage followed by the massage for the neck, shoulders and arms; the next day add the third section, and so on until you cover your body in one session.

Once you are familiar with the system it should be possible to complete the self-massage within fifteen minutes, but the movements should still be relaxed and never hurried. Doing the moves within this amount of time has an invigorating effect on the body. For a more relaxing effect perform the movements more slowly and take as long as you like to cover the whole body.

5 The moves

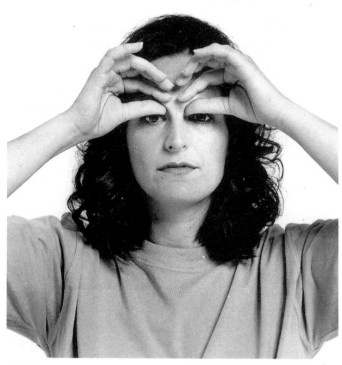

Fig. 1

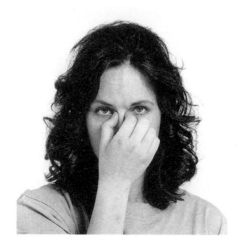

Fig. 2

There are certain massage 'moves' which you will need to become familiar with in order to do self-massage. These are used at different times during the massage sequence according to the part of the body being massaged. The moves (in order of appearance in the text) are:

Thumb and forefinger

Light massage to small areas and bony ridges, such as the eyebrows, is done by gently pressing with the thumbs and supporting with the inside edge of the lower part of the forefingers (Fig. 1).

Alternatively the thumb can be pressed against the ball of the index finger as in the massage of the bridge of the nose (Fig. 2).

Individual finger pressure

Pressure on acupoints or depressions between bones is given with a single finger, generally the middle or index finger or sometimes the thumb, while the rest of the hand is used as a support. The middle or index finger is used for the acupoints under the eyes (Fig. 3), sides of the ears, the cheeks, etc. The thumb is used for points on the elbows (Fig. 4), wrists, legs and back of the neck. Pressure is either vertical or in small, circular movements.

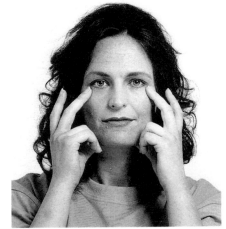

Fig. 3

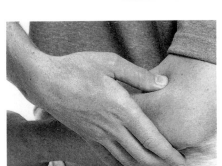

Fig. 4

Pressing a line

When massaging along a meridian line, such as the line of the Governor Vessel meridian across the back of the head, several fingers are used together to get good pressure (Fig. 5). The thumbs are used for support.

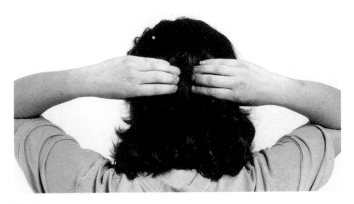

Fig. 5

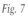

Fig. 6

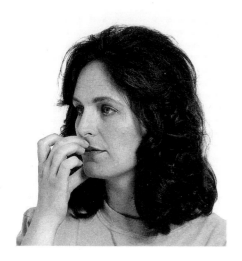

Nails

For sharp stimulation to a specific point, light pressure from the edge of the nail is used. The sensation should be stimulating but not painful. This is used for the point in the labial groove under the nose (Fig. 6) and for the insides of the ears.

Fig. 7

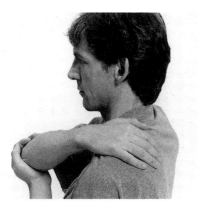

Palm squeezing

To apply pressure to a larger area, such as the shoulders, arms or legs, the open palm is first laid on the area and then squeezed in a rhythmical, flowing movement (Fig. 7). The fingers and the base of the palm, or the fingers and thumb, move in sequence with one another, and with each release the hand is moved slightly further along the limb or area of the body being massaged. The concentration should be on the releasing part of

Fig. 8

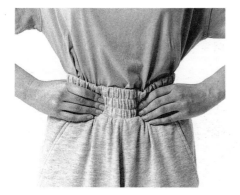

the movement rather than the squeezing. This technique is also used, with the hands at a slightly different angle, for the waist (Fig. 8).

Stroking

A 'stroking' technique is used for smoothing along the surface of the skin, or over clothing, on the shoulders (Fig. 9), abdomen and back. This simply involves gently smoothing the surface of the palm(s) over the area to be covered.

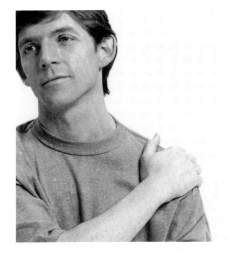

Fig. 9

Abdominal rotation

To apply firmer pressure to the abdomen, one hand is placed on top of the other and the two press into the abdomen simultaneously. Pressure is first applied with the fingertips, and then with the heel of the palm of the hand underneath.

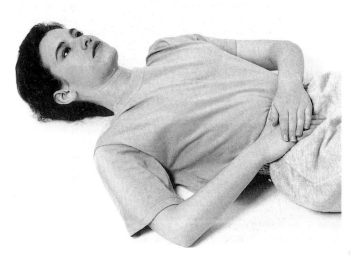

Fig. 10

Fig. 10 detail

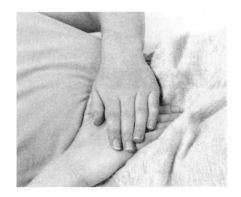

The movement is undulating, like a wave, and as much of the palm as possible is kept in contact with the abdomen (Fig. 10). As the hands massage they are slowly moved around the abdomen in a circle.

Elbows

Fig. 11

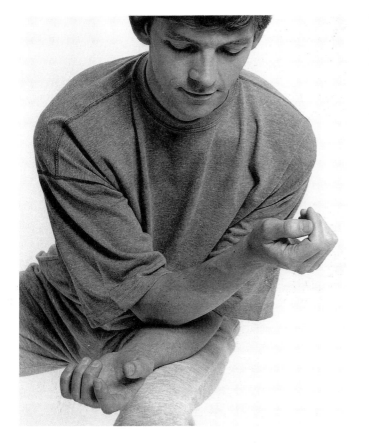

To apply more pressure to lower arms, palms or legs the elbows can be used (Fig. 11). First the elbow should be lightly placed in position, then weight is gradually leaned onto the elbow from the shoulders, chest and hips. Muscular force should not be used, just a transfer of weight to apply pressure. The hand and wrist should be relaxed, not clenched. Either the rounded or pointed edge of the elbow can be used according to the amount and type of pressure required.

Remember

- **All** pressure must be gentle and comfortable.
- Always start by **touching** – to make sure you are in the right position. Then **apply pressure**, starting gently and increasing until you have the firmness or stimulation you require. Then gradually ease off the pressure and **release**. Your movements should be a smooth sequence of TOUCH-PRESS-RELEASE with no sudden pressure or sharp movements.
- The whole body, especially the fingers and hands, should be relaxed during all the movements. If your hands, or any other part of your body, are tired or aching after the massage then you have been straining or maintaining tension. Keep checking you are relaxed throughout the massage until this becomes a habit.
- Keep your breath relaxed and free while applying self-massage and follow the breathing instructions given with each technique. Avoid the tendency to hold the breath while concentrating.
- The length of time the self-massage lasts depends on the effect you want to achieve. A brisk, quick massage in the morning is invigorating and stimulating and a good start to the day. A slower, more relaxed and flowing massage in the evening releases the day's tensions and prepares you for sleep.
- Always make sure some part of your body e.g. one of your fingers or one hand, is used for **support** while the other part(s) is being used for applying pressure. This ensures balanced touch and prevents painful or forceful pressure.
- **Intention** is important! Don't let your hands do the work while your mind wanders off onto something else. Mental worries will leave you tired and drained, while a clear mind, focused on the massage, will leave you refreshed. Use your mind to concentrate on each movement and add thoughts of peace and tranquillity with every touch.

SELF-MASSAGE

1 Warm-up

If you are going to carry out a complete self-massage, spend a few minutes preparing yourself first.

- Stop what you are doing, loosen any tight clothing and find a quiet place.
- Make yourself comfortable in a sitting or a lying position. Sit either in a chair with good back support or on the floor but with the back straight. Alternatively, lie on the floor or on a bed.
- Close your eyes and free your mind of thoughts so you can practise self-massage with a clear mind. If you wish, you can briefly review the day so far, or the day ahead, but see your thoughts passing in front of you as if on a film screen, and then let the screen go blank as your thoughts are released. If you find it hard to let your thoughts go completely, then mentally file them away to come back to later.
- Keeping your eyes closed, focus your attention briefly on your physical body. Note whether you feel tired or energetic, light or heavy, stiff or flexible. Observe areas of relaxation and any areas of tension, discomfort or pain. Decide which areas of your body may require special attention during the self-massage. Try to let any tension or tiredness slip away and allow your body to relax.
- Then turn your attention to your breathing. Allow your breathing to become deeper and more relaxed. Try breathing in through your nose and out through your mouth. Concentrate on the out-breath and let it be longer than the in-breath. Imagine that with each out-breath any stress, tension or tiredness is released, while with each in-breath new vigour enters your lungs and circulates throughout your body. If you wish, you can also add some breathing exercises (see page 107).
- After a few minutes of relaxed breathing, slowly open your eyes and stretch your whole body.
- Now do a few finger exercises to warm up your hands (see page 110).

You are now ready to begin your self-massage.

2 *The head and face*

Fig. 12

To start

Sit in a relaxed and comfortable position, either kneeling, cross-legged or in a chair. Rub the palms of your hands together and lightly run them up over your face and down the back of your head several times in a gentle, flowing movement (Fig 12).

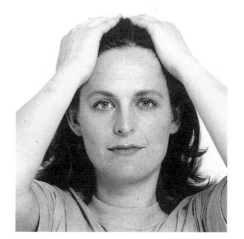

Eyes

Place your thumbs against the bony socket surrounding your eyes, by the bridge of your nose. Rest your forefingers on top of the edge of the bony sockets. Lightly press up with your thumbs against the bone and your forefingers (Fig. 13). The forefingers apply light pressure but are mainly used for support. Release the pressure and then move both thumbs and forefingers slightly outwards following the line of the bony socket. Again apply light

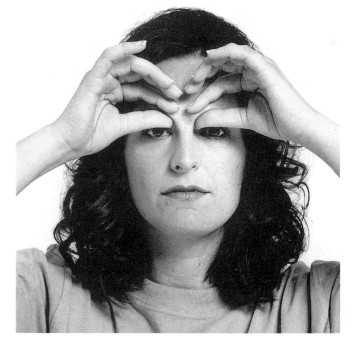

Fig. 13

Fig. 14

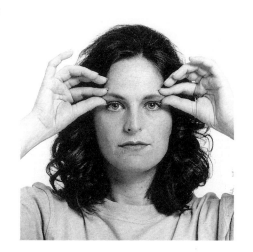

pressure and then release. Move your thumbs and forefingers outwards again and repeat the touch-press-release motion. Continue with this movement until you reach the outside of your eyes (Fig. 14).

Now change the positions of your hands. Use your thumbs to support your chin and then press lightly with your middle fingers against the bony socket underneath your eyes (Fig. 15). Slowly work along the lower sockets repeating the touch-press-release movement with your middle fingers until you reach the bridge of your nose and have made a complete circle around your eyes.

If you are doing a slow massage, exhale gently as you apply pressure and inhale as you release. Otherwise inhale as you work over the top of your eyes and exhale as you work underneath.

NOTE: Take care not to drag your fingers along the delicate skin around your eyes. Your fingers should be lightly released after each application of pressure and before

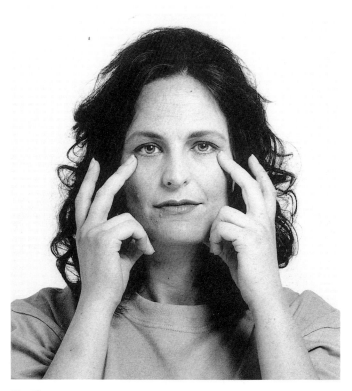

Fig. 15

moving on to the next position.

The complete movement around the eyes can be repeated several times if wished.

To finish the eye massage, rub the palms of your hands together and then gently rest them over your eyes with the heels of your palms over your eyelids and your fingertips on your forehead. This 'palming' technique has a very soothing effect on the eyes. Breathe deeply as you do this (Fig. 16).

Benefits: Helps to release tiredness and tension around your eyes.

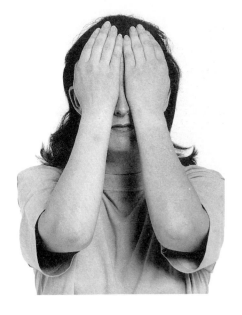

Fig. 16

Scalp

Place your fingers together in a line on the middle of your forehead. Rest your thumbs on your temples, at the side of your head, for support (Fig. 17). Apply firm but light pressure with your fingers only and then release. Lift your fingers slightly further up your forehead, towards

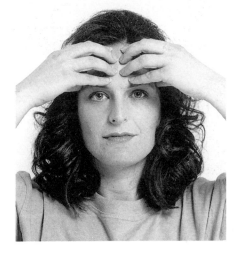

Fig. 17

Fig. 18

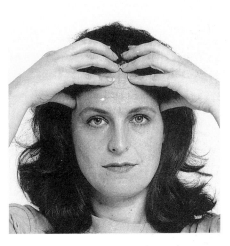

Fig. 19

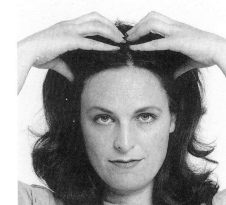

the hairline, raising your thumbs at the same time, and repeat the movement (Fig. 18). Continue this movement up and over the scalp (Fig. 19), following the line of the Governor Vessel meridian. When you reach the top of your head apply pressure at the acupoint Governor Vessel 20 (Fig. 20).

Acupoint Governor Vessel 20

Location: At the top of the head. Place the thumbs on the top of each ear and stretch the middle fingers to meet at the top of the head. The fingers should be on the mid-line, and the scalp in line with the nose.

Benefits: Improves mental function and general health. One of the major acupoints of the body.

Fig. 20

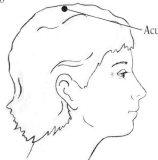

Acupoint: Governor Vessel 20

After massaging the acupoint GV20, continue pressing in a line along the centre of your scalp down to your back hairline moving your thumbs and your fingers simultaneously (Fig. 21). Then return to the front hair-line and repeat the same movement, this time with your fingers a half inch on either side of the mid-line of your head (Fig. 22). Once again use the touch-press-release movement with all your fingers working in a line from the front of your head, over your head and down to the hairline at the back of your head. Then repeat this movement once more, this time with your fingers one inch on either side of the mid-line (Fig. 23).

Synchronize the touch-press-release movements with your breathing. If you are doing a slow massage you can exhale as you apply pressure and inhale as you release. Otherwise do 1 or 2 complete movements to each inhalation and exhalation.

Fig. 21

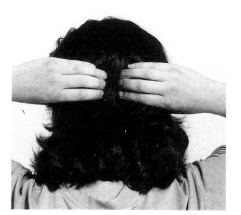

Fig. 22

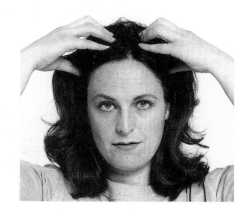

Fig. 23

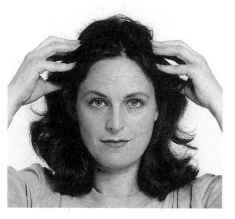

Benefits: Releases tension in your forehead and scalp. Stimulates mental function.

Fig. 24

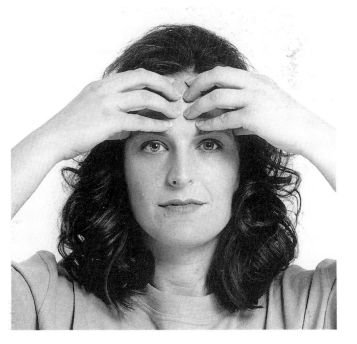

Forehead

Once again, place all your fingertips together in a vertical line on the middle of your forehead and let your thumbs rest against your temples for support (Fig. 24). Press lightly with your fingers and then release. Next, move your fingers about an inch apart. Touch your skin lightly then, again, press and release. Continue this movement until the whole forehead has been covered (Fig. 25).

Again, exhale as you apply pressure and inhale as you release or synchronize the movements with your breathing.

NOTE: Take care not to press too hard or this may give you a headache. Movements should always be with light, firm, comfortable pressure.

Fig. 25

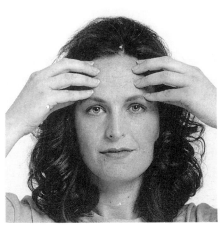

When you reach your temples, change the position of your hands so that your middle fingers rest on your temples and your thumbs rest on your jaw bone for support. Now gently massage your temples on both sides of your head by rotating your middle fingers upwards and backwards away from your eyes. Fit the rotations rhythmically to your breathing (Fig. 26).

Benefits: Releases tension in your forehead and temples. Relaxes your eye muscles.

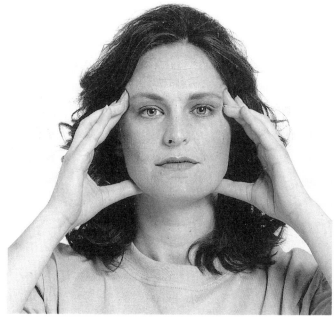

Fig. 26

Side of head

Keeping your thumbs in the same position, lower your middle fingers to just above your ears on either side of your head and continue to massage with gentle, circular movements (Fig. 27). Use the same movement to work with your fingers around the back of your ears to the acupoint Gall Bladder 20 (Fig. 28).

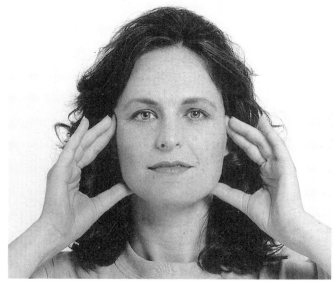

Fig. 27

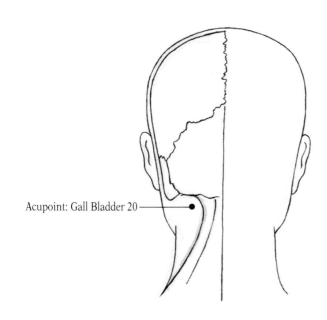

Acupoint: Gall Bladder 20 ——

Acupoint Gall Bladder 20

Location: At the back of the head in the depressions between the bottom of the skull and the large muscles of the neck.

Benefits: Releases neck tension and can ease headaches. Improves eyesight.

To massage this point rest your fingers on the back of your head and press into the point on each side of the neck with your thumbs. Again, use the touch-press-release movement, pressing lightly but firmly into the point. Alternatively, light, circular movements can be used. There should be a pleasant feeling of release of tension as this point is massaged. Breathe rhythmically and deeply as you apply the massage.

Benefits: Releases tension at the back of your head and neck and can ease one-sided headaches.

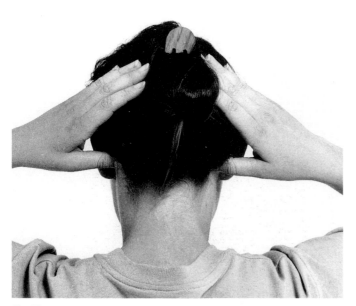

Fig. 28

Ears

According to oriental medicine, the ear represents a microcosm of the body and each part of the ear corresponds to a specific body part. The body is represented upside down on the ear, like a foetus in the curled position. For this reason the

1. Toe
2. Finger
3. Ankle
4. Wrist
5. Uterus
6. Knee
7. Pelvis
8. Buttock
9. Gall Bladder
10. Abdomen
11. Elbow
12. Urinary Bladder
13. Kidney
14. Pancreas
15. Lower Back
16. Large Intestine
17. Appendix
18. Small Intestine
19. Liver
20. Stomach
21. Chest
22. Shoulder
23. Oesophagus
24. Mouth
25. Spleen
26. Neck
27. Shoulder Joint
28. Trachea
29. Heart
30. Lung
31. Brain Point
32. Clavicle
33. Nose
34. Testis (ovary)
35. Forehead
36. Tongue
37. Eye
38. Internal Ear
39. Tonsil

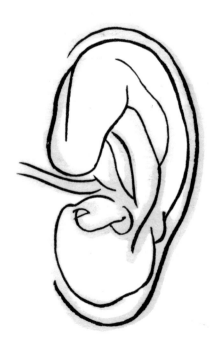

The ear (showing foetus position)

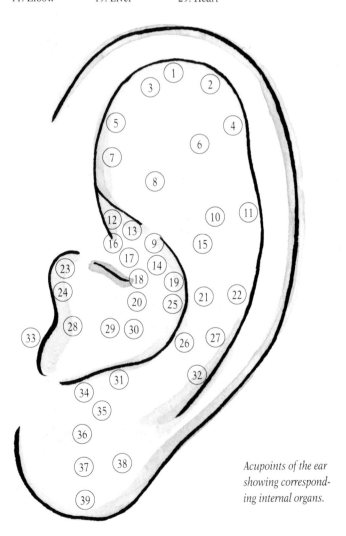

Acupoints of the ear showing corresponding internal organs.

Fig. 29

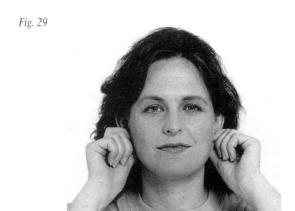

Fig. 30

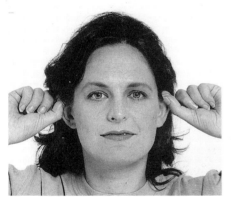

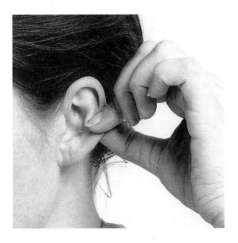

Fig. 31

ear is massaged from the base of the earlobe up to the top of the ear, as this maintains the principle of massaging the body from top to toe. Light stimulation of the many acupoints in the ear is said to tonify and strengthen each of the internal organs and body parts.

Begin with your earlobes, pressing your thumbs lightly against the tips of your forefingers (Fig. 29). Using the touch-press-release movement, work your way up along the outer edges of your ears. When you reach the tops of your ears, the position of your fingers can be reversed (Fig. 30). This outer part of your ear is said to correspond to the extremities of your body.

Return to your earlobes and repeat the movement, working from the bottom to the top, but this time with your fingers on the inside edges of your ears (Fig. 31). This part of your ear is said to correspond to your skeletal system.

Finally, take the edge of the nail of your index fingers and press lightly on the inside of your ears. Make sure that your nails are smooth and clean, and do not press too hard. This part of your ear is said to correspond to the inner organs of your body (Fig. 32).

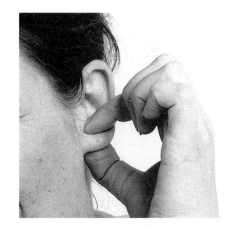

Fig. 32

Breathe normally throughout the massage.

Complete the ear massage by rubbing your hands back over your ears and then pulling them forward (Figs. 33 and 34). Inhale as you push your ears back, and exhale as you bring them forward. Repeat several times.

After this massage your ears will feel warm and tingling.

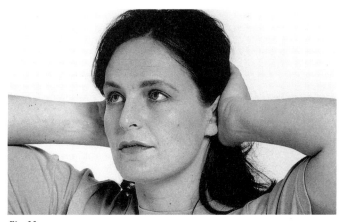

Fig. 33

Benefits: Massaging your ears releases tiredness and has a general stimulating effect on your body and mind. Also aids concentration and mental alertness.

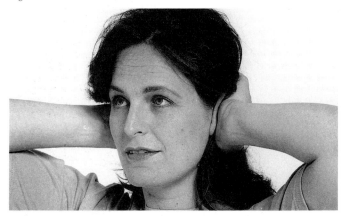

Fig. 34

Fig. 35

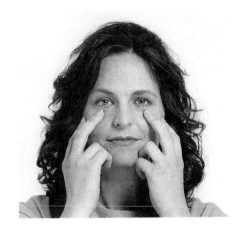

Cheeks

Rest your thumbs underneath your chin for support and press with your middle fingers against the acupoint Stomach 1 just below the eyes using the touch-press-release movement (Fig. 35).

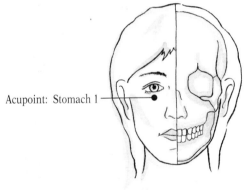

Acupoint: Stomach 1

Acupoint Stomach 1

Location: On the ridge of the bony cavity under the eye, directly below the pupil.

Benefits: Improves eyesight and balances digestion.

Next, lower your fingers to just beneath your cheekbones and repeat the touch-press-release movement (Fig. 36). Now work your way along the edge of your cheekbones out towards your ears, repeating the touch-press-release technique. If you wish, a slight circular rotation can be used with each movement. When you reach

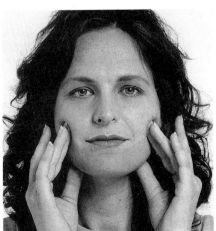

Fig. 36

the ears, massage the three acupoints at the front of each ear, i.e. Triple Heater 21, Small Intestine 19 and Gall Bladder 2.

Acupoint Triple Heater 21

Location: In the depression in front of the notch at the top of the ear. Locate with the mouth open (Fig. 37). *Benefits:* Eases tinnitus (ringing in the ears) and toothache.

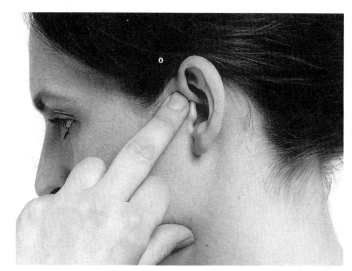

Fig. 37

Acupoint Small Intestine 19

Location: In the depression formed in front of the middle of the ear when the mouth is open (Fig. 38). *Benefits:* Eases tinnitus; helps maintain good hearing.

Acupoint Gall Bladder 2

Location: In the depression in front of the ear lobe when the mouth is open (Fig. 39). *Benefits:* Releases tension in the jaw; relieves toothache.

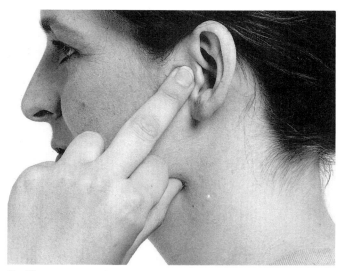

Fig. 38

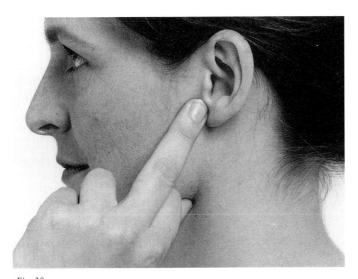

Fig. 39

For all the touch-press-release movements, exhale as you apply pressure and inhale as you release. Or, if you do not have time for this, apply a series of touch-press-release movements for the in-breath and then a series of movements for the out-breath.

Benefits: The cheek massage stimulates eyesight and hearing and promotes a good complexion.

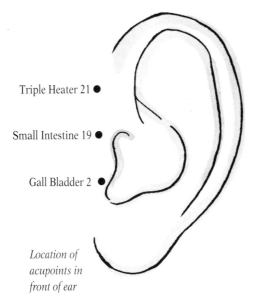

Triple Heater 21 ●

Small Intestine 19 ●

Gall Bladder 2 ●

Location of acupoints in front of ear

Nose

Lightly squeeze the bridge of your nose between the finger and thumb of one hand (Fig. 40). Then, gradually work down your nose using one hand, or the middle fingers of both hands (Fig. 41) until you reach your nostrils.

Use the touch-press-release movement or small circular rotations. If you are using both hands then have your thumbs on your chin for support. At the base of your nose apply direct stimulation to the acupoint Large Intestine 20, located on either side of each nostril, using small circular rotations (Fig. 42).

Acupoint Large Intestine 20

Location: In the groove just below the outside edge of each nostril.
Benefits: Clears sinuses and nasal congestion.

Next, using the nail of your middle finger on one hand, press lightly in the groove just below your nose on the acupoint Governor Vessel 26 (Fig. 43).

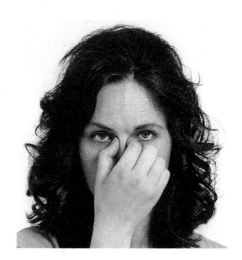

Fig. 40

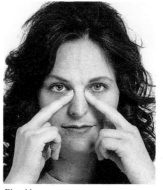

Fig. 41

Fig. 42

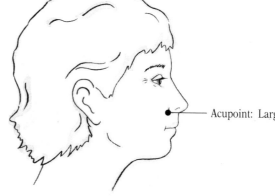

Acupoint: Large Intestine 20

Fig. 43

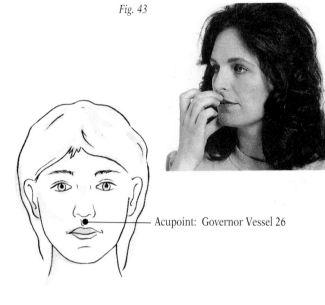

— Acupoint: Governor Vessel 26

> **Acupoint Governor Vessel 26**
>
> *Location:* In the groove directly below the nose.
> *Benefits:* Relieves faintness and improves concentration. Eases pain in your lower back.

As before, exhale as you apply pressure and inhale as you release.

Benefits: Clears your nasal passages and stimulates the senses.

Fig. 44

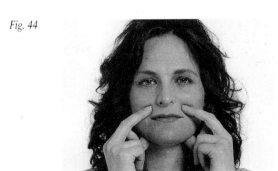

Fig. 45

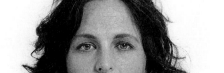

Mouth

Supporting your chin with your thumbs, press with your middle or index fingers around the top of your lips out to the corner of your mouth, using the touch-press-release movement (Fig. 44). Then massage under your lower lips until your fingers meet at the centre of your chin (Fig. 45). Again, exhale as you apply pressure and inhale as you release, or do a series of movements with each breath.

Now rest the arms and use the tongue tip to massage along the gums in a circular movement, three times in one direction and then three times in the other (Fig. 46).

Benefits: Improves the health of your gums and stimulates the production of saliva which is important for digestion.

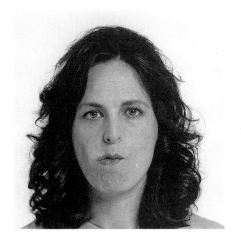

Fig. 46

Jaw

Use your thumbs for support underneath your chin (Fig. 47) and place your middle fingers in the jaw tension-release point (Gall Bladder 2) in front of your earlobe (see page 36). Massage down your jaw using circular, tension-releasing movements (Fig. 48). Now massage underneath your jaw by placing your fingers on your chin for support and then pressing inwards and upwards under the jawbone with your thumbs (Fig. 49). Work in lines from the outside of the

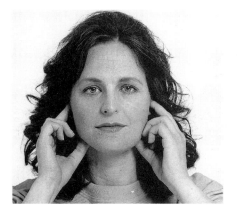

Fig. 47

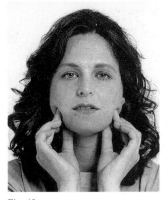

Fig. 48

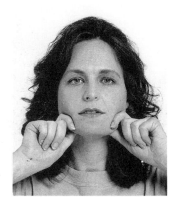

Fig. 49

Fig. 50

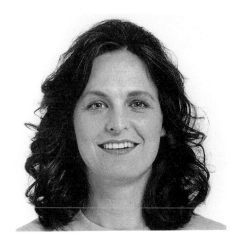

jawbone in towards the chin and synchronize your breath with the movements.

To complete this massage, relax the arms, open the mouth into a wide smile and release (Fig. 50). Repeat this movement three times.

Benefits: Releases tension in the jaw; eases sore throats and toothache.

Fig. 51

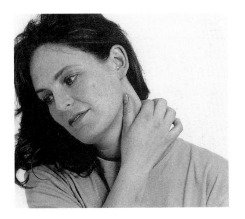

Neck

Turn your head slightly to one side. Place your thumb and forefinger of one hand on either side of the large muscle (the sternocleido-mastoid) at the side of your neck (Fig. 51). Massage from the top of the muscle down to the bottom by pressing the thumb lightly against the ridge of your forefinger and using the touch-press-release movement (Fig. 52). Return to the top of the muscle and repeat the massage down along the length of the muscle several times. Then turn

Fig. 52

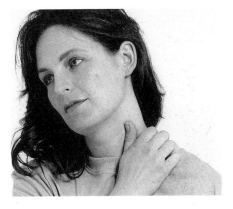

your head over to the other side and repeat the sequence using the opposite hand to massage the muscle on this side of the neck (Fig. 53). Each massage down to the base of the neck should constitute one breath.

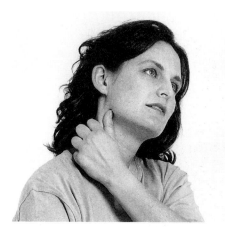

Fig. 53

If wished, the muscles on both sides of your neck can be massaged simultaneously (Fig. 54).

Benefits: Releases neck tension; eases sore throats.

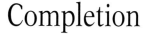

Completion

Rub the palms of your hands together once more and, again, lightly move them up over your face and then over the back of your head and neck (Fig. 55). This time, alternate your hands and repeat the movement several times. Inhale as you smooth up over your face, and exhale as you smooth down over the back of your head and neck (Fig. 56). The movements should be slow and relaxed.

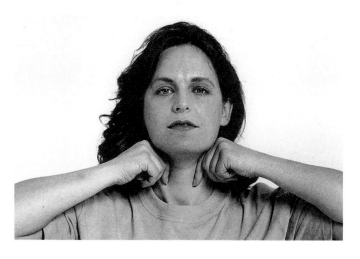

Fig. 54

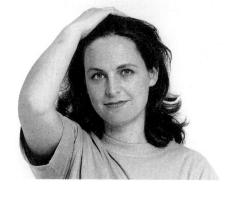

Fig. 55

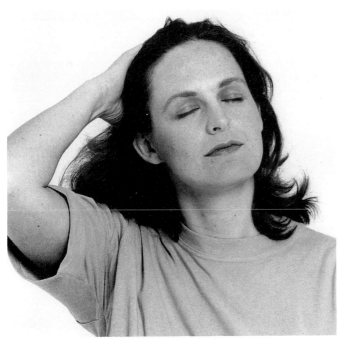

Fig. 56

If you wish, the palms can again be rubbed together and the palming technique (laying the palms over the eyes) can be repeated in order to relax and refresh your eyes further (see page 26).

If your arms get tired during this massage, then many of the movements can be performed whilst supporting your elbows on a table. At the end of the massage your whole face should feel tingling and refreshed and your skin should be glowing.

3 *The neck, shoulders and arms*

To start

If continuing on from the head and face massage, stay in the same position as before and continue with the massage. Change your position if it becomes uncomfortable.

If starting this section independently, then adopt a comfortable position either seated in a chair, or on a stool, or on the ground with the legs outstretched or cross-legged; whatever feels most natural for you (Fig. 57).

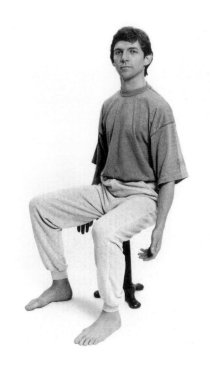

Fig. 57

Back of neck

Place your fingers over the back of your head with your thumbs resting on either side of your cervical vertebrae (neck bones) on the hairline (Fig. 58). Press in with your thumbs and then release. Repeat this touch-press-release movement, working outwards with your thumbs along the hairline until you reach

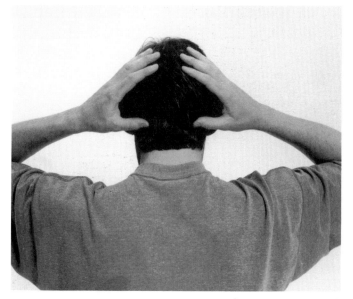

Fig. 58

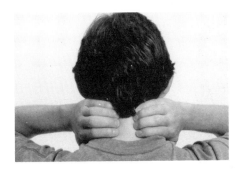

Fig. 59

Fig. 60

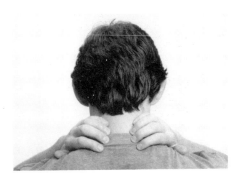

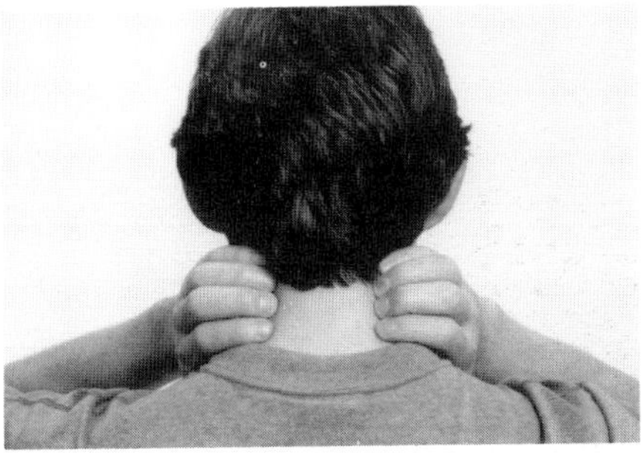

Fig. 61

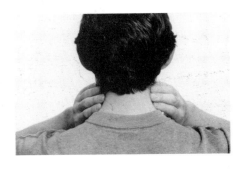

Fig. 62

your ears. Next, place your hands around the side of your neck, and this time rest your fingers on either side of the neck vertebrae (Fig. 59).

Slowly work down the sides of your vertebrae using the touch-press-release movement or light circular rotations until you reach the base of your neck (Fig. 60). Take care not to press on the bones themselves, just on either side of them.

Return to the top of your neck, but this time place your fingers half an inch further out on each side (Fig. 61). Then repeat the touch-press-release movement, or circular rotations, down to the base. Finally, repeat once more, this time with your fingers on the sides of your neck (Fig. 62).

Breathe normally and synchronize your breath with the movements. If you are doing a slow massage you can exhale with every application of pressure and inhale with each release.

Benefits: Releases tension in the back of your neck; increases circulation to your head.

Shoulders

Support your right elbow in your left hand and place your right hand over your left shoulder (Fig. 63). Starting close to your neck, use the palm-squeezing technique (see chapter on massage moves, page 17) to move down and out across your shoulder. This involves first placing your palm over your shoulder, close to your neck, then gripping the large muscle over your shoulder blade (the trapezius) by gently squeezing your fingers against your palm (Fig. 64). Breathe in as you do this. Then, as you breathe out, release your grip and slide your palm a little further down your shoulder to the next position. Repeat the palm-squeezing technique. Work all the way down to the edge of your shoulder (Fig. 65) and then repeat the complete movement from the base of your neck out to your shoulder two or three times.

Remember that the emphasis for

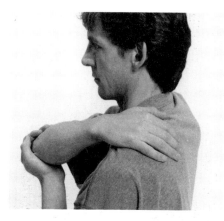

Fig. 63

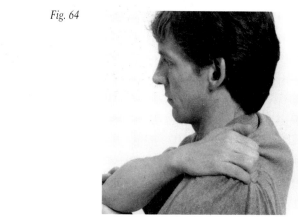

Fig. 64

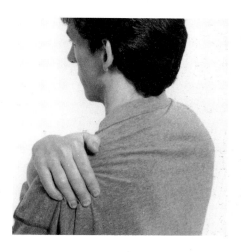

Fig. 65

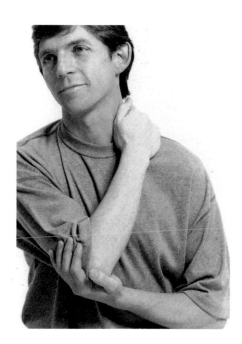

Fig. 66

this movement is on the releasing action rather than the squeezing, as the aim is to release any tension or stiffness.

Follow this by repeating the entire sequence on your opposite shoulder, taking care to support your elbow to prevent your arm getting tired.

Finish off by stroking down each shoulder with the flat of the opposite palm. Breathe in as you raise your palm and place it on your shoulder by your neck (Fig. 66). Then breathe out as you do a series of strokes to the edge of your shoulder (Fig. 67). Imagine that with each stroke you are wiping away any remaining tension.

At the end of this massage, your shoulders should feel tingling and relaxed.

Benefits: Releases tension in your neck and shoulders. Relieves stiff necks and eases tension headaches.

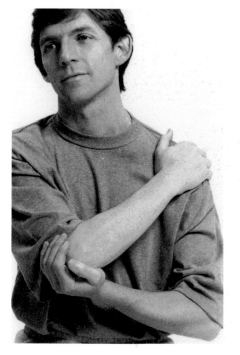

Fig. 67

Underarms

Raise your left arm slightly and rest your right hand under your left armpit with your thumb in front (Fig. 68). Use a gentle, squeezing movement between your thumb and fingers working down and then back up your armpit (Fig. 69). Then repeat on the opposite side. Take care to use very gentle movements around your armpits, especially if the area is tender. Do one squeezing technique for each inhalation and exhalation.

Benefits: This massage stimulates lymphatic drainage and eases shoulder stiffness or pain.

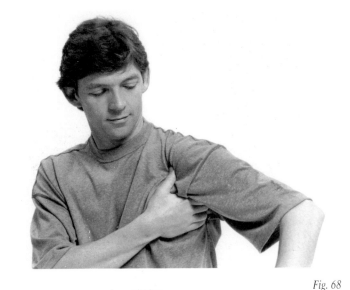

Fig. 68

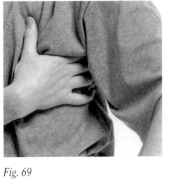

Fig. 69

Arms

The massage described here goes through the complete massage for the left arm and then repeats the procedure for the right arm. This is generally the easiest and most com-

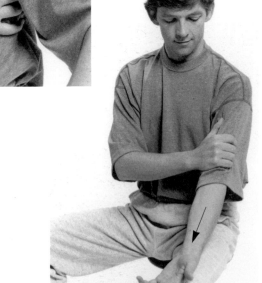

Fig. 70

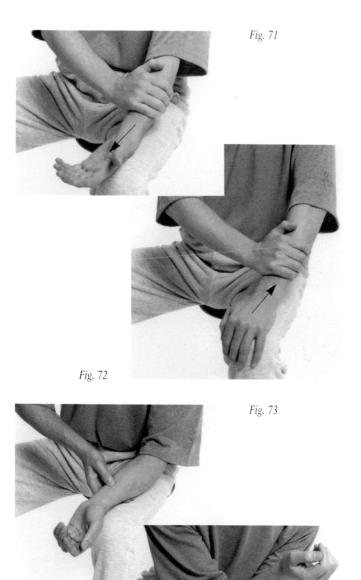

Fig. 71

Fig. 72

Fig. 73

Fig. 74

fortable way to practise the massage. Alternatively, if preferred, each movement can be done first on one arm and then on the other, working through both arms simultaneously.

Keeping your left arm raised or resting it on the thigh, begin to massage down from your armpit along the inside of your upper arm to your elbow (Fig. 70). Use the same gentle palm-squeezing technique, and then continue on down your forearm to your wrist (Fig. 71). Next, turn your hand over and work in the same way up your outer arm from your wrist up to your shoulder (Fig. 72). Synchronize your breathing with the movements.

On your forearm it may be easier to apply pressure with your thumb, using your palm for support (Fig. 73). Alternatively, firm pressure may be applied using the elbow (Fig. 74).

It is important to massage **down** the **inside** of your arms and **up** the **outside** of your arms, as this follows the direction of flow of the meridians in the arms.

Make sure that while doing this massage your shoulders are relaxed, your back straight and that you are breathing freely. If you are doing a slow, relaxed massage you can time each movement with the breath (i.e. breathe in as you squeeze with your palm and breathe out as you release).

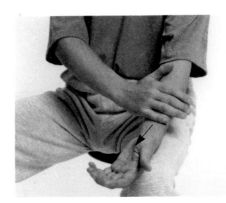

Fig. 75

To complete the arm massage, stroke down the inside of your left arm (Fig. 75) and up the outside (Fig. 76) with the palm of your right hand. Breathe out as you stroke down and inhale as you stroke up to your shoulder.

Benefits: Releases tension in the arms; eases stiff shoulders, stimulates your arm meridians.

Fig. 76

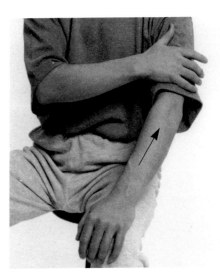

Fig. 77

Elbow

When you reach your elbow, as you are massaging up your outer arm, stop to massage the acupoint Large Intestine 11 (Fig. 77).

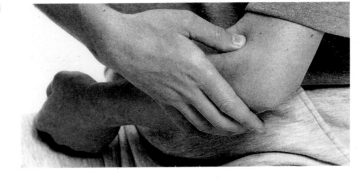

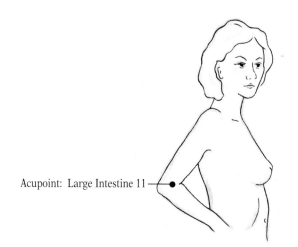

Acupoint Intestine 11

Location: At the end of the elbow crease when the arm is bent.

Benefits: Eases stiffness or pain in the elbow; aids digestion; relieves constipation.

Acupoint: Large Intestine 11

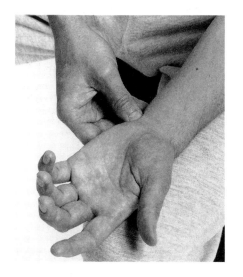

Fig. 78

Wrists

Stroke down the inside of your left arm once more to return your right hand to your wrist. A circular massage is now performed around your wrist in order to free the wrist bones and stimulate important acupoints in this area.

Start on the inside of your wrist, pressing downwards with your thumb into the acupoint Heart 7. For this movement your left wrist is supported by the fingers of your right hand and your thumb presses in with a gentle, rotating movement directed towards your palm (Fig. 78).

Acupoint Heart 7

Location: On the inside crease of the wrist, level with the little finger.

Benefits: Eases chest pain, palpitations, irritability, and insomnia.

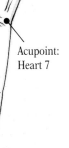

Acupoint: Heart 7

Next, continue to massage around the skin crease on your wrist, known as the 'bracelet' of the wrist, until your thumb is located in the middle of your wrist between the two small tendons (Fig. 79). These tendons can easily be seen if your wrist is flexed backwards and forwards. This is the location of the acupoint Pericardium 7. Make several rotations with your thumb into this point, keeping your fingers underneath for support.

Continue massaging with your thumb a little further around the bracelet of the wrist until you reach the acupoint Lung 9 (Fig. 80). Again, apply several light rotating movements into this point in the direction of the thumb.

Acupoint Pericardium 7
Location: In the middle of the wrist crease between the tendons.
Benefits: Relieves cardiac pain, nausea, car sickness and feelings of anxiety.

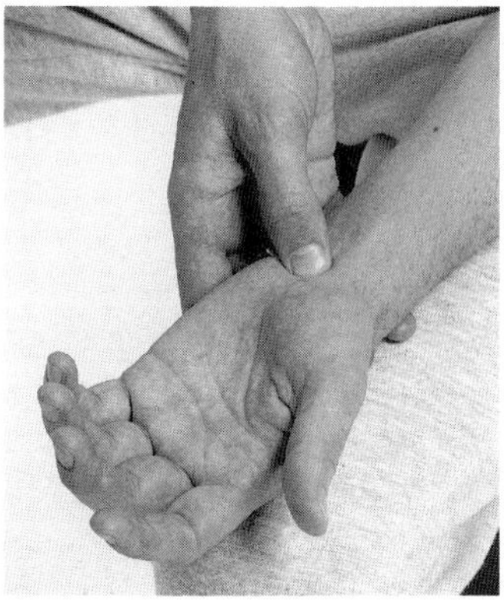

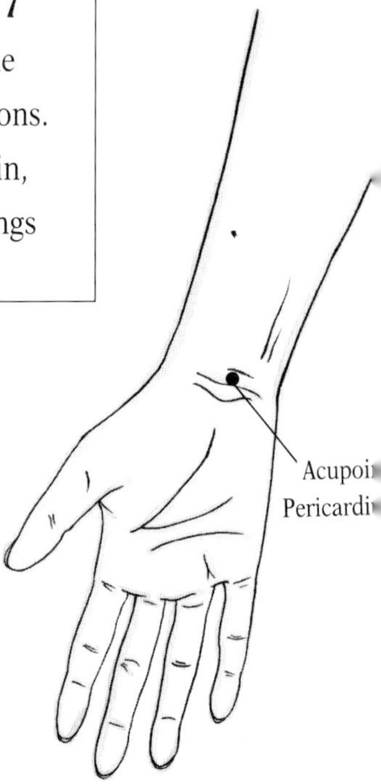

Fig. 79

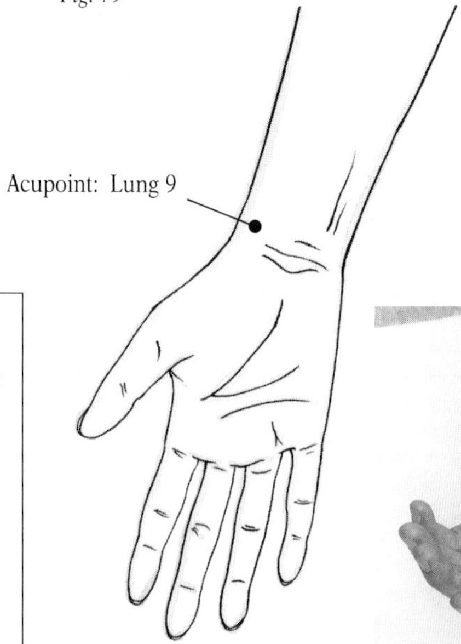

Acupoint
Pericardi

Acupoint: Lung 9

Fig. 80

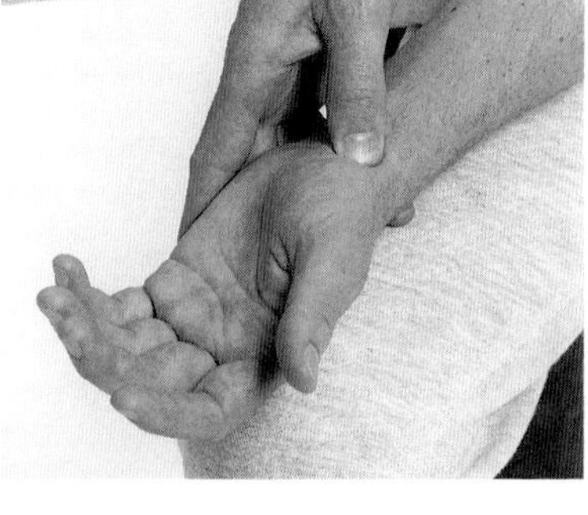

Acupoint Lung 9
Location: On the crease of the wrist in the depression in line with the thumb.
Benefits: Strengthens the lungs. Relieves asthma, sore throats and chest pain.

Now turn your left hand over and place your right hand over the back of it. Keep your right thumb in contact with your wrist as you slide your hands round. As your thumb slides round your wrist it should come to rest on the acupoint Large Intestine 5. Make several rotations into this point, pressing in the direction of your elbow (Fig. 81).

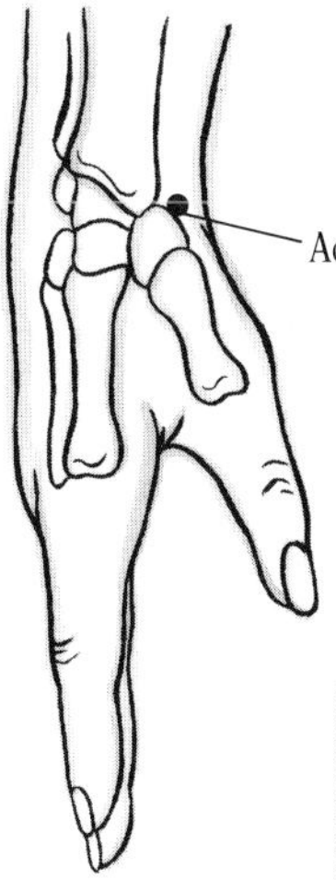

Acupoint: Large Intestine 5

Acupoint Large Intestine 5
Location: On the upper side of the wrist in the depression between the tendons when the thumb is lifted. *Benefits:* Relieves wrist pain, headaches, sore throats, toothache and sore eyes. Promotes a good complexion and strengthens eyesight.

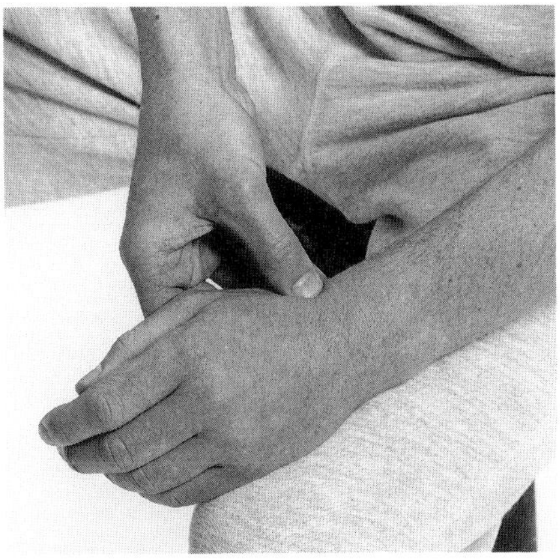

Fig. 81

Continue massaging with your thumb around the top of your wrist until you reach the depression in front of the bone on the outer side of your wrist where the acupoint Triple Heater 4 is located. Massage into the point with the thumb angled slightly in the direction of the elbow (Fig. 82).

Acupoint Triple Heater 4

Location: In the depression between the bones of the hand (the metacarpals) and the head of the bone on the outside of the arm (the ulna), in line with the ring finger.
Benefits: Relieves pain or stiffness in the wrist, shoulder and arm. Helps increase circulation in the hands.

Finally, move your thumb and right hand around further until your thumb is pressing into the depression on the outer edge of your wrist where the acupoint Small Intestine 5 is located. Make several rotations with your thumb angled slightly towards your elbow (Fig. 83).

Acupoint Small Intestine 5

Location: In the depression between the bones on the outer side of your wrist.
Benefits: Eases wrist and neck pain; helps to release shoulder tension.

This completes the circular massage around your wrist. Maintain normal,

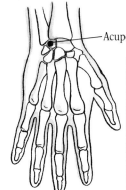

Acupoint: Triple Heater 4

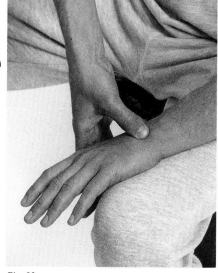

Fig. 82

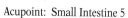
Acupoint: Small Intestine 5

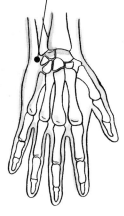

Fig. 83

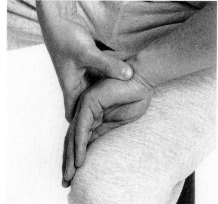

rhythmical breathing throughout
this part of the massage and make
sure your neck and shoulders remain
relaxed and your back straight
throughout.

Benefits: Increases mobility of your
wrist. Relieves stiffness or pain in
your wrists. Stimulates important
acupoints around your wrist.

Acupoint Large Intestine 4

Location: In the centre of the
triangle made by the metacarpal
bones of the index finger and thumb.
Benefits: A general tonic point for
the whole upper body; improves
complexion and aids digestion.

Hands & Palms

First massage the acupoint Large
Intestine 4, in between the index
finger and thumbs, on your left
hand. Then turn your hand over,
supporting it with the fingers of
your right hand. Press with your
right thumb into the lower part of
the palm in line with your little
finger. Make small rotations with
firm pressure (Fig. 84).

Fig. 84

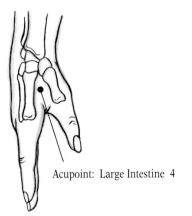

Acupoint: Large Intestine 4

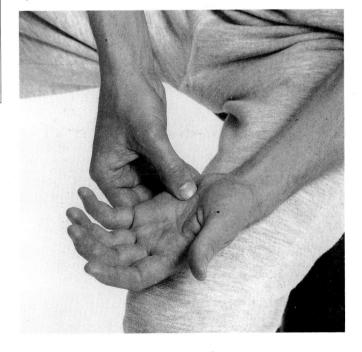

Working in a clockwise direction, use your thumb to massage around your palm in a circle. Use the touch-press-release movement, or small rotations. When you reach the top of your palm, concentrate on the fleshy spaces in between the bones (Fig. 85).

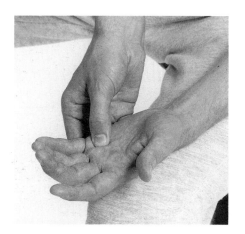

Fig. 85

When the circle around your palm has been completed, slide your thumb into the centre of your palm on the acupoint Pericardium 8 (Fig. 86). Massage deeply with your thumb using your fingers below as support.

Fig. 86

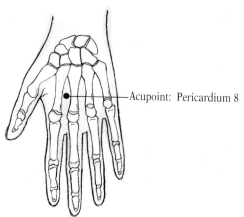

Acupoint Pericardium 8

Location: In the centre of the palm between the bones. At the point where the middle finger touches the palm when it is bent forward.
Benefits: Relieves anxiety, nausea and chest pain. Helps freshen the breath.

Breathe normally while massaging your palm and keep your fingers relaxed.

Benefits: Keeps your hands mobile. Relieves aching hands; calms your mind.

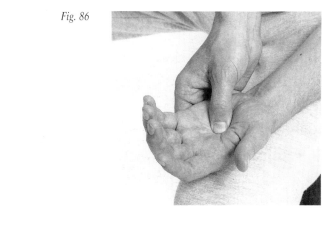

Acupoint: Pericardium 8

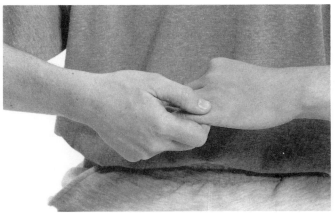

Fig. 87

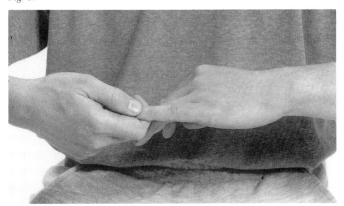

Fig. 88

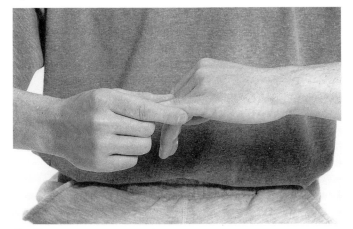

Fig. 89

Fingers

Take the base of your left hand little finger between the thumb and forefinger of your right hand. The thumb should be on top of the finger, and the edge of the index finger below (Fig. 87). Pressing between your thumb and forefinger, massage down your little finger to the nail tip (Fig. 88). Pull slightly on the finger as you do this.

Return to the base of your little finger, and now place your thumb and forefinger on either side of it (Fig. 89). Again massage down the finger to the nail tip by using touch-press-release movements.

Repeat the same movement for each of the fingers of your left hand, working from the little finger to the thumb. Take special care to massage the edges of the nail beds on each finger as these are the location of the starting and ending point of each of the meridians in the arms. Massage of these points has a powerful effect on the flow of energy within the meridians.

Maintain normal breathing, or, if you wish, you can breathe out as you massage down each finger, completing your exhalation as you reach the nail tips, and inhale as you return to the base of each finger.

Completion

Shake your wrist out loosely (Fig. 90). Make a fist and rotate your wrist five times in each direction (Fig. 91). Keep your shoulders straight and elbow still. You can also add some of the finger exercises here (see page 110).

Benefits: Increases mobility of your fingers. Can relieve stiffness and certain types of arthritic pain.

Opposite arm

Now repeat the entire sequence for the right arm.

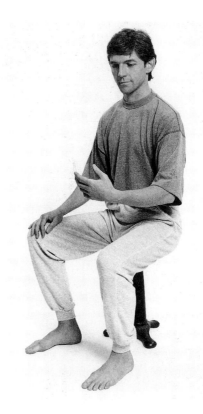

Fig. 90

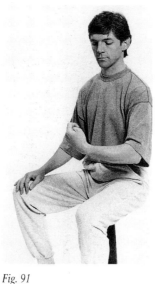

Fig. 91

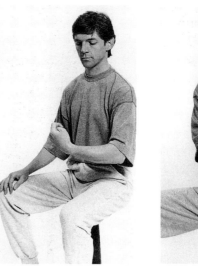

Fig. 92

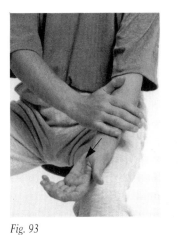
Fig. 93

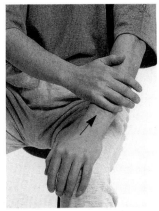
Fig. 94

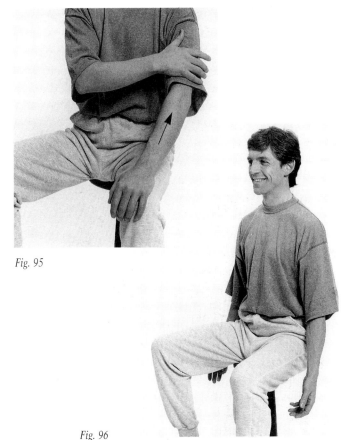
Fig. 95

Fig. 96

Completion

Shake your hands out and rub your palms together. Breathing in, place the palm of your right hand over your left shoulder, close to your neck and stretch your left arm out, palm uppermost (Fig. 92). Exhaling, smooth your palm over your shoulder and down the inside of your arm, all the way to your fingertips (Fig. 93).

Then, inhaling, turn your left arm over (Fig. 94) and smooth up the outside of the arm to your shoulders (Fig. 95). Breathe out and relax your arms by your sides (Fig. 96).

Inhale once more and place your left palm over your right shoulder while stretching out your right arm with your palm uppermost. Then repeat the procedure for your right shoulder and arm. If you have time, breathe normally in the final position for a few minutes, with your eyes closed if you wish.

This completes the massage of your neck, shoulders and arms.

4 *The chest and abdomen*

To start

If you are continuing on from the previous sections you can stay in the same position. If starting with this section, sit in a relaxed position and breathe quietly for a few minutes. Visualize the body and internal organs as healthy and energetic.

Throat

Rest your thumbs on the collarbone for support and then press the middle fingers lightly against the end of the collarbone nearest your throat. Take care to press against the ridge of the bone rather than into the throat itself. Work around the edge of the bone using the touch-press-release movement. Breathe normally and keep your shoulders relaxed and your back straight (Fig. 97).

Benefits: Relaxes your throat; helps relieve sore throats.

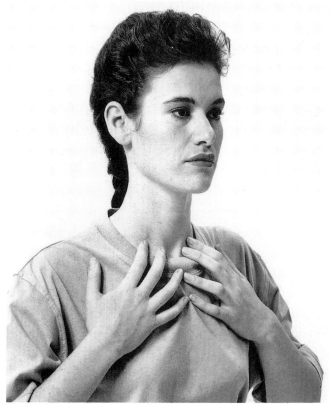

Fig. 97

Fig. 98

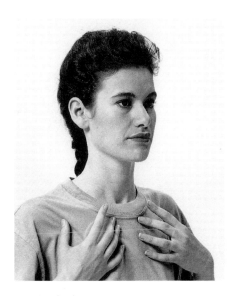

Fig. 99

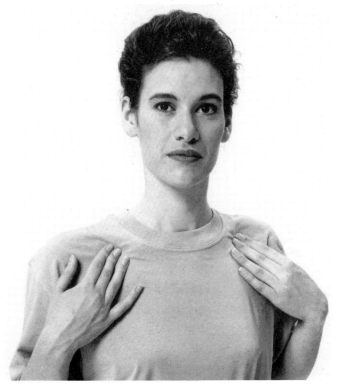

Collarbone

Move your middle fingers down below your collarbone (Fig. 98). Massaging just below the collarbone, work outwards with your fingers from the centre of the chest to your shoulders using the touch-press-release movement (Fig. 99).

You can massage with either your index or middle fingers, or both can be used together. The supporting thumbs are moved outwards as necessary.

Repeat the movement along the length of your collarbone, moving from the centre of the chest to the sides, several times. Breathe freely as you do so and keep your shoulders relaxed and back.

Benefits: Helps to 'open' your chest. Relieves colds and congestion of the lungs.

Breastbone (sternum)

Resting your thumbs in your armpits (Fig. 100), press with your middle fingers on either side of your breastbone in the middle of your chest (see the skeletal system diagram in the Appendix). Start at the top by your throat and slowly work down on either side of your sternum to the middle of your chest (Fig. 101). Use the touch-press-release movement or small rotations. When you reach your mid-chest, massage the acupoint Conception Vessel 17.

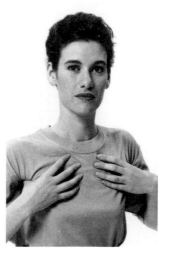

Fig. 100

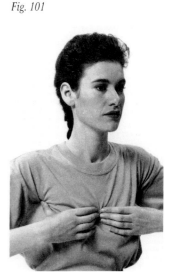

Fig. 101

Acupoint Conception Vessel 17

Location: In the middle of the chest and breastbone, in line with the nipples.
Benefits: Relieves asthma, hiccoughs and chest pain. Strengthens the lungs and heart.

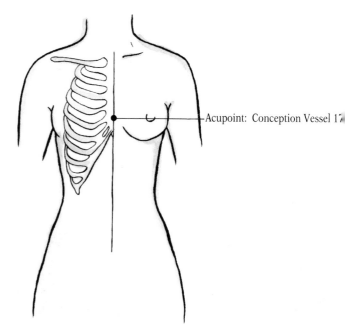

Acupoint: Conception Vessel 17

If doing a slow, relaxed massage, inhale as you locate your fingers and exhale as you apply pressure. Otherwise, breathe normally.

Benefits: Strengthens the lungs. Helps prevent and relieve all types of respiratory problems.

Rib-cage

Keeping your thumbs under your armpits for support, return your middle fingers to the top of the sternum. With these fingers, locate the space between your top two ribs (Fig. 102). Massage along this space from your breastbone out to your shoulders using the touch-press-release movement (Fig. 103).

Return your fingers to your breastbone and locate the space between your next two ribs. Repeat the massage out to the sides (Fig. 104). Continue in this way working along the space between each rib, down to the bottom of the rib-cage.

Fig. 102

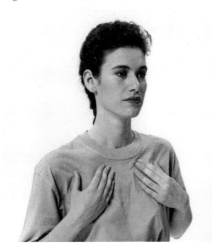

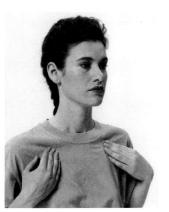

Fig. 103

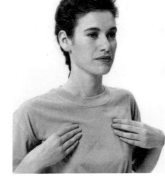

Fig. 104

Make sure to accurately follow the line of your ribs out to the sides of your body and take care not to press too hard on your lower ribs, which can be quite fragile. Again, either breathe normally or exhale each time pressure is applied, and inhale as you release.

NOTE: For women – first massage your top ribs then carry out breast massage, as shown below, and finally work along your lower ribs (Fig. 105).

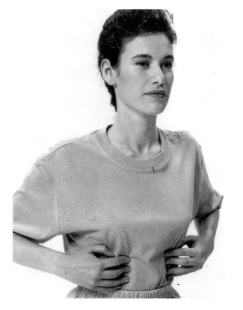

Fig. 105

Breast Massage

Place your left hand behind your neck, or on your shoulder, and raise the elbow. Massage gently around your breast using the soft pad of the finger tips of your right hand (Fig. 106). Massage first underneath your breast then out to the sides and round over the top (Fig. 107). Use light, gentle rotation movements and breathe in as you work up and round your breast and out as you work down the inside.

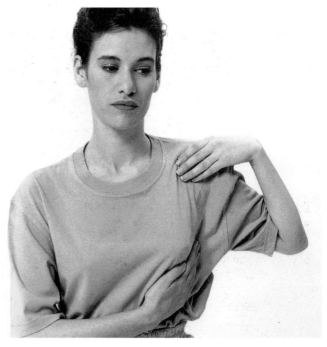

Fig. 106

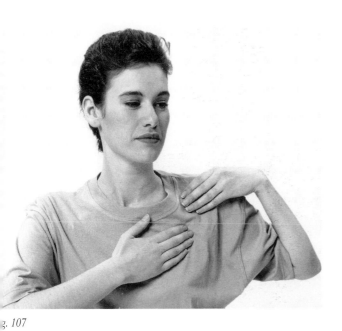

*. 107

Repeat on the other side.

If you practise breast self-examination (leaflets on this can be found in any health centre or Well Woman Clinic) this can be incorporated into the massage.

Follow this by massaging your lower ribs as described above.

Benefits: Massage of your rib-cage releases tension in your chest and facilitates deep breathing. Breast massage helps to firm and tone your breasts.

Fig. 108

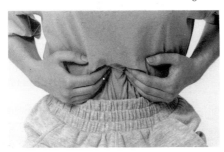

*. 109

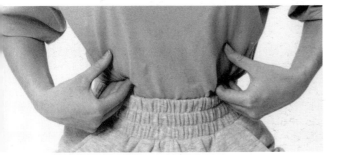

Under ribs

Gently hook the fingers of each hand underneath your ribs (Fig. 108). Then massage from the centre of your body out to your sides using the touch-press-release movement to press gently up and under your ribs (Fig. 109). Breathe out each time you apply pressure, and in as you release. This will make the movement more comfortable and enable you to press in deeper under your ribs. If you wish, this movement can be performed standing up.

Benefits: Releases epigastric tension; aids digestion.

Abdomen

Waist Squeeze

If you are seated on a chair you will need to sit forward in order to perform this movement, or else stand up. If seated on the floor you may wish to come up to a kneeling position or else lie down.

Place your hands around your waist with your thumbs behind (Fig. 110). Press in deeply with your fingers and thumbs and use a squeezing movement to massage your waist (Fig. 111). Repeat a rhythmical squeeze and release movement several times. Breathe in as you squeeze with your hands, and out as you release.

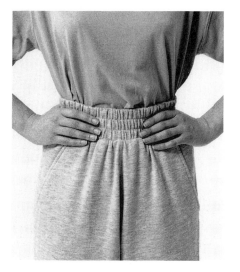

Fig. 110

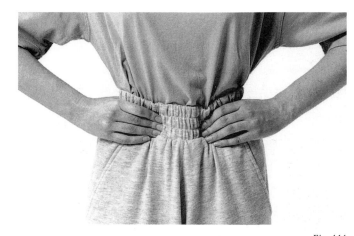

Fig. 111

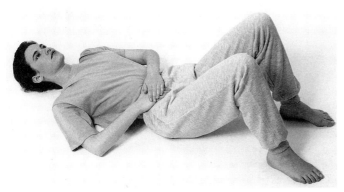

Fig. 112

Abdominal Rotation

This movement is best performed lying down on the floor, or on a firm mattress, with your knees bent.

Place your right palm on the lower right side of your abdomen and rest your left hand on top (Fig. 112). Press into the abdomen with both hands using an undulating movement starting with your fingers and working through to the heel of your palm. The movement is a gentle rocking made by your right hand with your left hand as support. Press in quite deeply but gently (Fig. 113).

As your hands perform the rocking massage they are gradually moved up and around the abdomen in a circular movement following the line of the Large Intestine (see Appendix 3). That is, they are moved up to just below the waist (Fig. 114), across the abdomen just below the navel (Fig. 115), down the left side of the abdomen (Fig. 116) and finally, over the pubic bone back to the starting position.

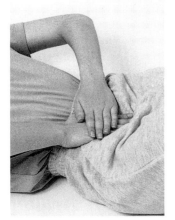

Fig. 113

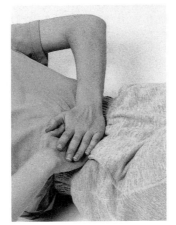

Fig. 114

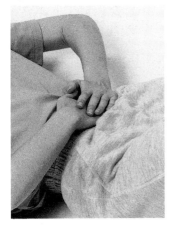

Fig. 115

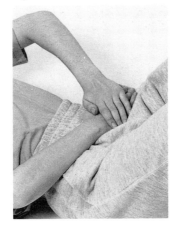

Fig. 116

The whole circular movement can be repeated several times. With deep breathing this is a very relaxing technique. Breathe out as you apply pressure into your abdomen, and in as you release.

Benefits: Regular massage in this way aids digestion, releases abdominal tension and can relieve constipation.

Stroking

Repeat the above movement with one hand on top of the other but this time lightly smooth the surface of your abdomen rather than pressing in deeply (Fig. 117). Continue to move in circles around your abdomen in a gradually decreasing spiral until your two palms end up in the centre of your abdomen (Fig. 118). Breathe in as you smooth up and over your abdomen, and breathe out as you smooth down.

This point, in the centre of your abdomen, is known in Japanese as the 'Tanden'. In oriental medicine this is said to be the central source of energy in the body.

Benefits: Calms your emotions and develops confidence.

'Heavenly peace'

When you reach the 'Tanden' point, rest with your hands there for a few minutes, close your eyes and breathe deeply.

Benefits: Calms body and mind.

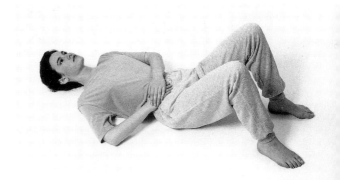

Fig. 117

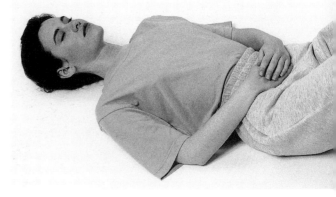

Fig. 118

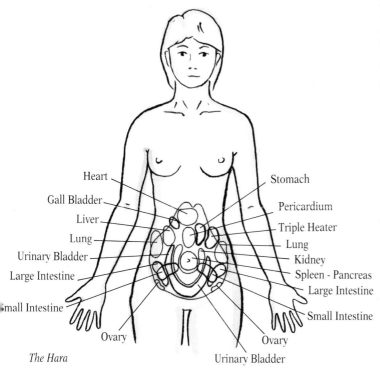

Heart
Gall Bladder
Liver
Lung
Urinary Bladder
Large Intestine
Small Intestine
Ovary

Stomach
Pericardium
Triple Heater
Lung
Kidney
Spleen - Pancreas
Large Intestine
Small Intestine
Ovary
Urinary Bladder

The Hara

Hara

In oriental medicine the abdominal area is known as the 'Hara'. Like the ears, the 'Hara' is said to be a microcosm in which each of the vital organs is represented (see diagram). Hara massage is a specialist technique used in oriental medicine for both diagnosis and treatment of the internal organs. The technique takes many years to perfect. However, even the simple abdominal massage described above can help to tone and balance each of the internal organs.

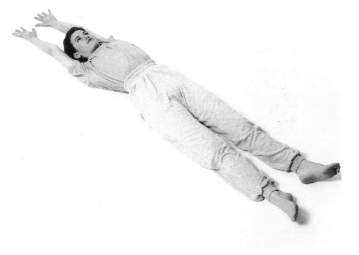

Fig. 119

Completion

You can stay relaxing in the 'Heavenly Peace' position for as long as you like. When you have finished, stretch your legs out and your arms up above your head as you inhale and open your eyes (Fig. 119). Exhale as you lower your arms to your sides.

This completes the massage of your chest and abdomen.

5 *The back*

To start

If you are continuing on from the previous section, bend your knees once more (Fig. 120), drop them over to one side (Fig. 121), roll over onto all fours (Fig. 122) and sit up (Fig. 123). Stay in this kneeling position or stretch your legs out in front of you.

If starting with the back massage, you can sit on a chair or stool, or on the floor either kneeling or with your legs stretched out in front.

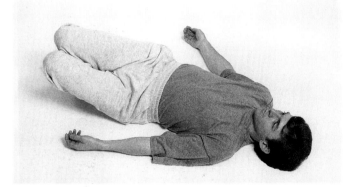

Fig. 120

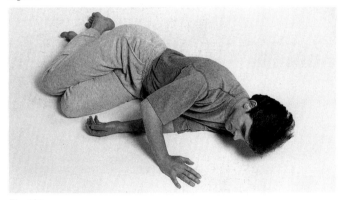

Fig. 121

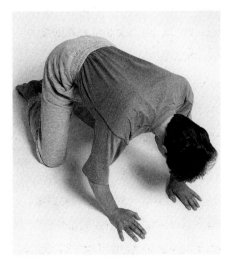

Fig. 122

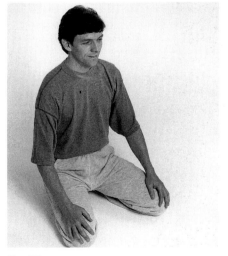

Fig. 123

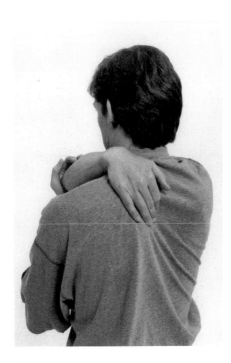

Fig. 124

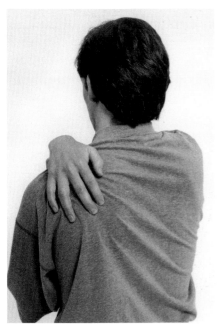

Fig. 125

Shoulder blade (scapula) massage

Support your right elbow in your left hand and place your right palm over the back of your left shoulder (Fig. 124). Use the palm-squeezing technique to massage the large muscle (the trapezius) which covers your shoulder blade (scapula). (See Appendices 1 and 2 for diagrams of the muscles and bones.) Squeeze the muscle firmly and then release. Work rhythmically from your neck out towards the edge of your shoulders (Fig. 125). Inhale as you squeeze the muscle and exhale as you release.

Next, raise your elbow slightly higher enabling your hand to move a little further down your upper back. Continue to massage from your spine out to your sides, this time using your fingertips and the touch-press-release movement, working across your shoulder blade.

Exhale as you apply pressure with your fingers, inhale as you release.

Finish by lightly pummelling over the same area with a flat palm (Fig. 126) and then by smoothing with stroking movements as you breathe normally.

Repeat the complete sequence on the opposite side.

Benefits: Releases tension in your shoulders and upper back.

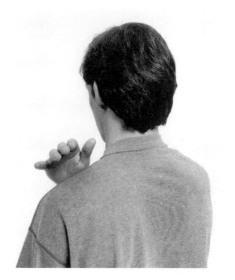

Fig. 126

Middle back

Place your hands around your middle back with your thumbs at your sides for support. Have your hands as high up your back and rib-cage as comfortably possible. Press with your middle fingers on either side of your spine (Fig. 127). Do not press on your spinal bones (vertebrae) themselves. Locate the spaces between your ribs at the back and massage with your fingers along these spaces, moving from your

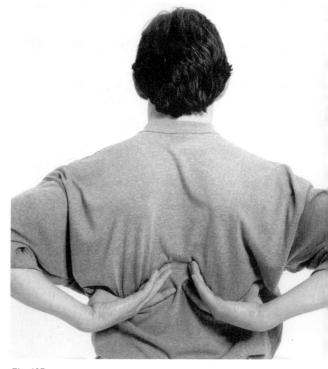

Fig. 127

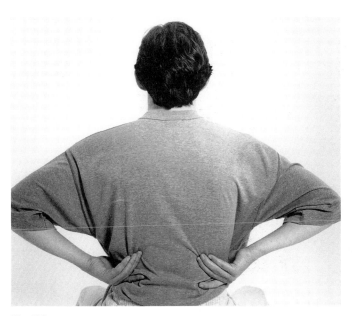

Fig. 128

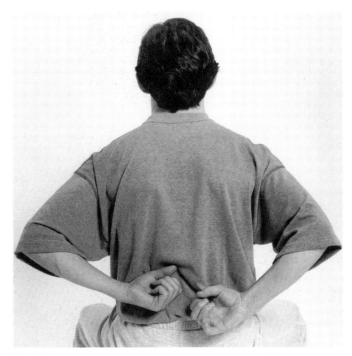

Fig. 129

spine out towards the sides of your body (Fig. 128). Use the touch-press-release movement and apply gentle but firm pressure. Pay special attention to the areas of the kidneys just below your ribs (see Appendix 3). If doing a slow massage, exhale as you apply pressure and inhale as you release. Otherwise, breathe normally.

Benefits: Releases tension in your back; stimulates kidney function.

Pummelling

Next, shake your arms out loose, relaxing them for a moment. Then make loose fists with your hands and use these to pummel gently over the areas of the kidneys (Fig. 129). Take care not to pummel too hard. This movement should be invigorating and refreshing and not painful or uncomfortable. Breathe normally.

Benefits: A good 'pick-you-up' when you feel tired. Helps to expel toxins via the kidneys and leaves you feeling refreshed.

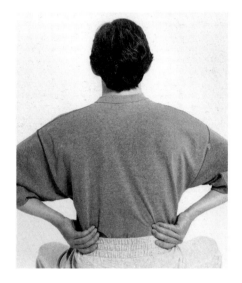

Fig. 130

Lower back

Place your hands around your waist with your thumbs in front (Fig. 130). Apply the palm-squeezing technique to massage the whole of your lower back and buttocks (Fig. 131). Either inhale as you squeeze and exhale as you release, or breathe normally.

If you wish, you can also use individual finger pressure to release pain or tension on sensitive spots (Fig. 132). In this case, breathe out as you apply pressure and breathe in as you release.

Benefits: Relieves pain and tension in your lower back and hips. Aids healthy menstrual function in women.

Fig. 131

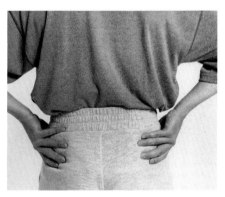

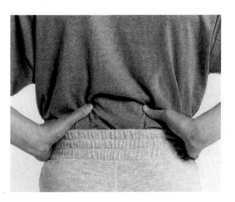

Fig. 132

Knuckle position

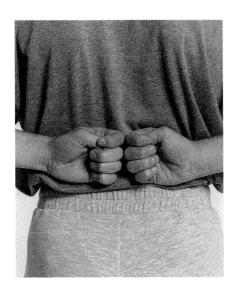

Knuckle pressure

To apply deeper pressure to your middle and lower back, lie flat on the floor, with your knees raised, and place your loosely clenched fists on either side of your spine, with your knuckles uppermost. Don't press against your spine itself but just on either side of it.

Start with your fists as high up your back as is comfortable and press with your back into your knuckles as you exhale (Fig. 133). Then, inhaling, transfer your weight onto your feet, raise your back slightly, and move your knuckles an inch further down the floor (Fig. 134). Again exhale as you lower your back gently onto your knuckles, which should now be level with the next vertebra (Fig. 135). Continue in this way massaging down your back on either side of your spine.

Finally, return your knuckles to your upper back and place them

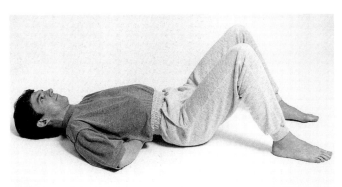

Fig. 133

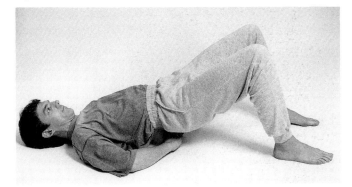

Fig. 134

slightly further out to your sides.
Repeat the massage sequence
working down to your lower back.
The knuckle pressure can also be
used to massage your buttocks.

Benefits: Releases tension in your
lower back and hips. Tones the back
muscles.

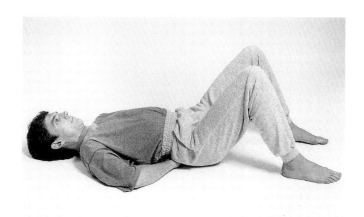

Fig. 135

Spinal massage aids

If you have difficulty reaching each
of the bones of your spine, you may
find a simple massage device
helpful. Wooden rollers, available at
health shops, can be placed on the
floor and gradually worked along
the length of the spine. Alternatively,
two tennis balls wrapped in a sock
can be used. Place them on the floor
with one ball on either side of the
spine. Lower your upper back onto
the balls. Have your legs bent and
your feet flat on the floor. Push with

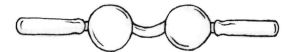

your feet in order to edge your back slowly over the balls. Move very slowly, inching down your spine.

Spinal roll

To apply gentle massage to the whole of your spine, sit on the floor and then grasp your knees, either underneath or in front (Fig. 136). Gently rock backwards and forwards (Fig. 137) stimulating each part of the spine.

NOTE: For comfort you can do this on a soft surface such as a blanket or some folded towels. Breathe out as you roll back and inhale as you roll forwards.

Benefits: Strengthens your back and tones your muscles.

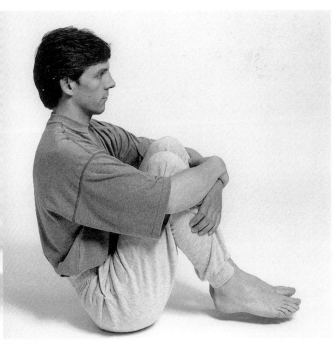
Fig. 136

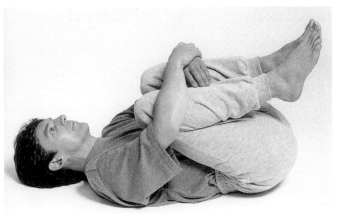
Fig. 137

Spinal Stretch

Lying flat, stretch your arms over
your head and point your toes,
breathing in as you do so (Fig. 138).
Imagine drawing breath into each of
the bones of your spine and filling
and expanding the spaces between
them. As you exhale, lower your
arms to your sides once more and
relax your body completely. Repeat
the movement several times.

Benefits: Stretches your spine and
promotes relaxation.

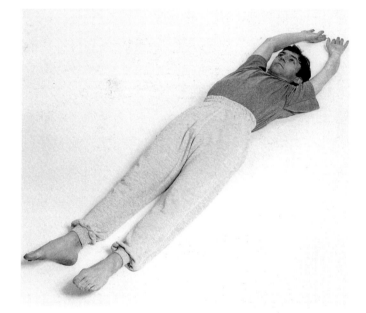

Fig. 138

Spinal twists

Spinal twists may be performed
lying down or sitting up in order to
strengthen your spine and the
muscles around each of the vertebrae.

Lying down

Lie flat on the floor with your arms
outstretched, palms facing down-

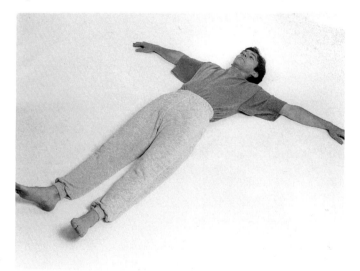

Fig. 139

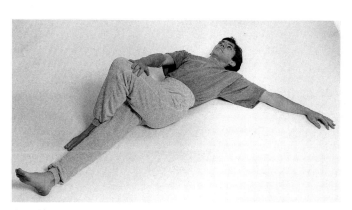

Fig. 140

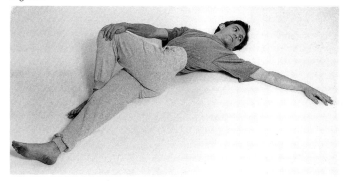

Fig. 141

wards and legs straight (Fig. 139). Place your left foot against the outside of your right knee as you inhale (Fig. 140). Keeping your arms out to the sides and your shoulders flat on the ground, exhale as you gently lower your left knee towards the ground, stretching your spine as you do so (Fig. 141). If you wish you can use your right hand to gently pull the left knee to the floor, but keep the left shoulder flat on the floor. Hold this position for a moment, breathing normally. Next, inhale as you return your knee to the upright position, and then exhale as you stretch your leg back out.

Repeat the movement with your other leg.

NOTE: Take care to keep your shouldders flat on the ground in order to get the correct stretch of your spine. It is more important to have the shoulders in the correct position than to try to force the knees down to the floor. As the back becomes more supple, the knee will naturally move more easily to the floor.

Sitting position

Stretch your right leg out in front of you, and place your left foot on the outside of your right knee (Fig. 142). As you inhale, place your right hand on the outside of your left knee, and your left hand behind you. Now, exhaling, slowly turn to look over your left shoulder, twisting and stretching your spine as you do so (Fig. 143). Hold for a moment, breathing normally, and then slowly return to the starting position on an exhalation.

Repeat on the other side.

Benefits: Increases flexibility of your spine; firms your back muscles; trims your waist.

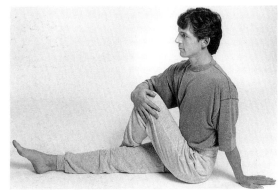

Fig. 142

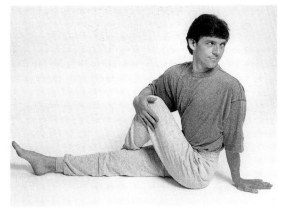

Fig. 143

Acupoints

In oriental medicine the back is also a microcosm for the body as a whole. All along your back there are acupoints which correspond to your internal organs. With back massage these acupoints are stimulated, helping to tonify and balance each of your internal organs, as well as strengthening your back itself.

A lot of tension is stored in your back and shoulders. Massage of these areas releases it, leaving you feeling relaxed and refreshed.

This completes the back massage.

The legs and feet

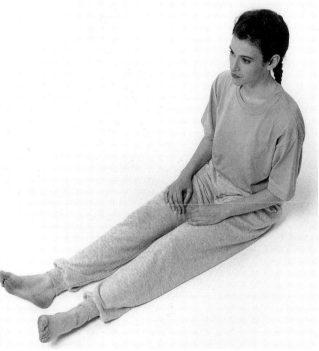

Fig. 144

To start

Sit comfortably on the floor with your legs stretched out in front of you. Adjust your heels so that they are in line with one another and your hips straight. Keep your back upright and breathe normally (Fig. 144).

As with the arm massage, your legs can be massaged either one by one, or movement by movement on one leg after the other. The description below is for the complete massage of one leg at a time

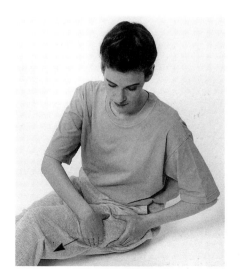

Fig. 145

Thighs

Place your left and right palms side by side over the top of your left thigh. Massage down the outside of your thigh (Fig. 145) to your knee using either the squeeze technique – grasping your thigh with your palms and squeezing with your fingers and thumb in a rhythmical movement –

or pressing in a line with your thumbs (Fig. 146), using your fingers as support. When you reach your knee, move your hands over to the inside of your thigh. Now work back up the inside of your thigh (Fig. 147) and continue massaging up to your groin area.

Now place your fingers round the back of your thigh with your thumbs at the sides for support (Fig. 148). Massage down the back of your thigh to the back of your kneecap, pressing in a line with your fingers and using your thumbs as support.

It is important to massage **down** the **outside** of your thigh, **up** the **inside** and **down** the **back** in order to follow the direction of the flow of the meridians. You can bend your leg slightly if you find this easier.

NOTE: For firmer pressure your left elbow may be used (Fig. 149). To do this correctly, place the soft edge of your elbow along your thigh, gently lean your weight onto your elbow to apply pressure, and then release.

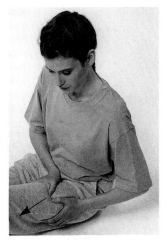

Fig. 146

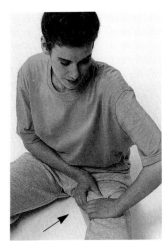

Fig. 147

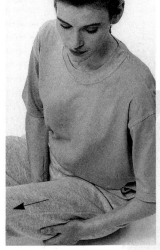

Fig. 148

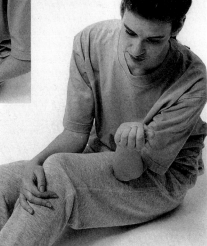

Fig. 149

Benefits: This increases circulation in your thighs and stimulates your leg meridians.

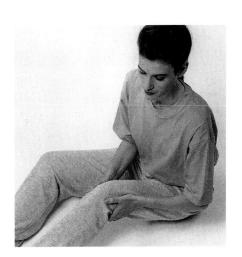

Fig. 150

Knees

Bending your knee, place your thumbs around your kneecap (patella), and your middle fingers behind your knee (Fig. 150). Press up into the back of your knee using the touch-press-release motion. First press into the centre of the back of your knee. Then move your fingers out on either side of the tendons at the back of your knee. These are easier to locate when your knee is bent.

Next, use your thumbs to massage the front of your kneecap, keeping your fingers at the back of your knee for support. First, massage in the two depressions at the top of your knee and then the two just below your knee (Fig. 151, 152). Synchronize your breathing with the movements.

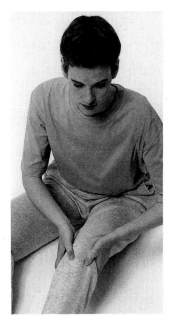

Fig. 151   *Fig. 152*

Knee acupoints

Location: These points are located in the depressions just above and below the kneecap.

Benefits: Eases knee joint pain; relieves stiffness in the knees.

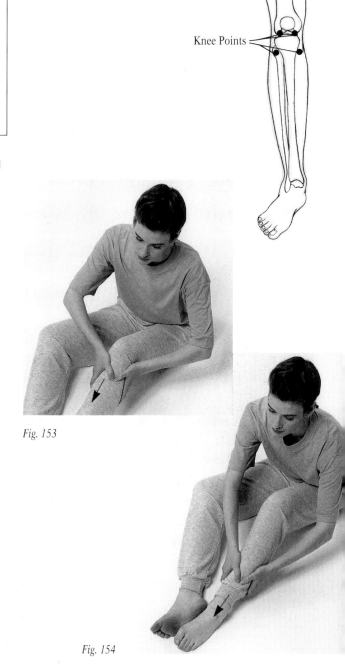

Knee Points

Lower Legs

Bending your left leg a little further, place your thumbs on the outside of your leg, just below your knee joint, and rest your fingers and palms on the sides of your leg for support (Fig. 153). Now apply pressure with your thumbs, using the touch-press-release movement and supporting with your fingers. Continue to massage down the outside of your leg in this way, as far as your ankle bone (Fig. 154).

You can also use the palm-squeezing technique or elbow pressure if you wish.

As you massage down your leg, pay special attention to the Stomach 36 point.

Fig. 153

Fig. 154

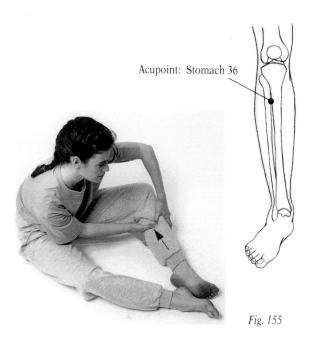

Acupoint: Stomach 36

Fig. 155

> **Acupoint Stomach 36**
> *Location:* Three fingers below the knee in the depression between the bones.
> *Benefits:* Relieves indigestion, diarrhoea, constipation and nausea.

When you reach your ankle, move your hands around to the inside of your ankle and then massage up the inside of your leg to your knee (Fig. 155). Again, use one or other of the techniques described above.

Finally, place your thumbs in front of your knee and your fingers behind your kneecap (Fig. 156). Then work down the back of your lower leg using either the squeezing technique or pressing in a line with your fingers using your thumbs as support (Fig. 157).

Benefits: This eases tired and aching legs; relieves cramp and strengthens digestion.

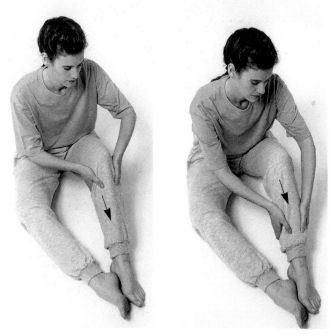

Fig. 156   *Fig. 157*

Ankles

As with the wrists, a circular rotation is made around your ankles using the touch-press-release movement and small rotations to massage important acupoints. Try to keep your thumbs in contact with your ankles when your arm or leg positions are changed.

Raise your left ankle towards your right thigh and place your arms on the inside of your left leg. Support your ankle with your fingers and use your thumbs to press into the acupoint Kidney 3 using the touch-press-release technique (Fig. 158).

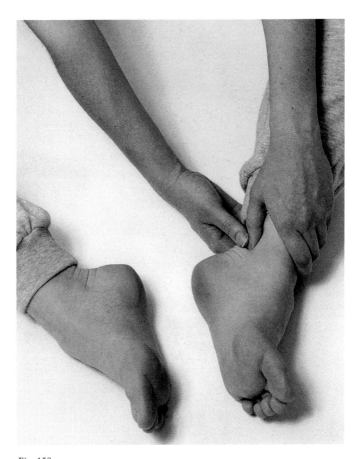

Fig. 158

Acupoint Kidney 3

Location: On the inside of the ankle in the depression level with your ankle bone.

Benefits: Relieves sore throats, toothache, ear problems, irregular menstruation and low back pain.

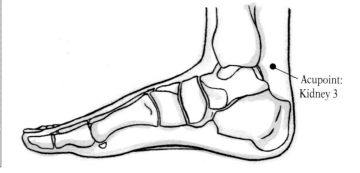

Acupoint: Kidney 3

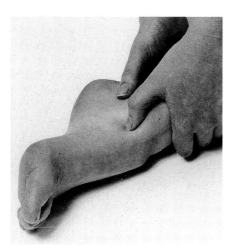

Fig. 159

Continue to massage in a circular direction around your ankle, under the ankle bone and round to the acupoint Spleen 5 (Fig. 159).

Acupoint Spleen 5

Location: In the depression between the ankle bones in line with the big toe.
Benefits: Relieves pain in the foot and ankle, aids digestion.

Then continue to massage over to the acupoint Liver 4 (Fig. 160).

Acupoint Liver 4

Location: In between the tendons at the front of the ankle.
Benefits: Promotes health of the gynaecological organs.

Now straighten your left leg and place your left arm on the outside of your leg. Keep your right thumb in contact with your ankle as you do so. Then locate the next acupoint around your ankle, Stomach 41, and apply small rotational pressure to the point (Fig. 161).

Acupoint: Spleen 5

Acupoint: Liver 4

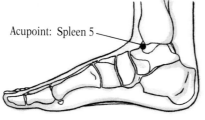

Fig. 160

Acupoint Stomach 41

Location: Between the tendons level with the tip of the ankle bone.
Benefits: Eases frontal headaches, dizziness and vertigo; relieves constipation and abdominal distension.

Keeping contact with your left thumb, now bend your leg over with your knee towards your thigh, and place both arms on the outside of your leg. Continue to massage around your ankle until you reach the next acupoint, Gall Bladder 40 (Fig. 162).

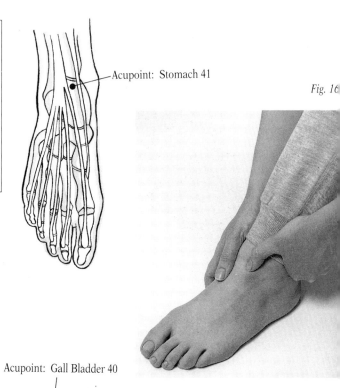

Acupoint: Stomach 41

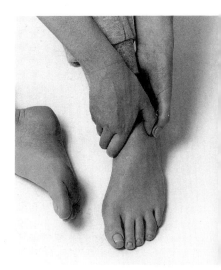

Fig. 16

Acupoint Gall Bladder 40

Location: On the outside of the ankle bone on the outer edge of the tendon.
Benefits: Strengthens the lower extremities; and tones the muscles.

After massaging the acupoint Gall Bladder 40, continue slightly further around the outside edge of your ankle to the acupoint Urinary Bladder 60 (Fig. 163).

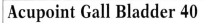

Acupoint: Gall Bladder 40

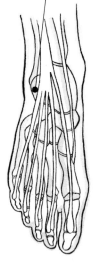

Fig. 162

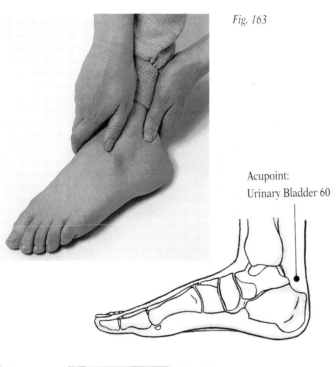

Fig. 163

Acupoint:
Urinary Bladder 60

Acupoint Urinary Bladder 60

Location: In the depression behind the ankle bones at the back of the ankle.

Benefits: Strengthens urinary function; relieves neck and low back pain, eases neck tension; improves eyesight. Increases mobility of your ankles and stimulates the flow of energy in your leg meridians.

NOTE: If the ankle massage is difficult with your leg bent, try straightening your leg a little and bending further from your waist.

To complete the ankle massage, place the index finger of your left hand on the Urinary Bladder 60 point, on the outside of your ankle, and your thumb on the Kidney 3 point, on the inside. Massage by rotating your finger and thumb in small circular movements towards the back of your ankle (Fig. 164).

Then stretch your legs out and gently rotate your ankles several times in both directions (Fig. 165).

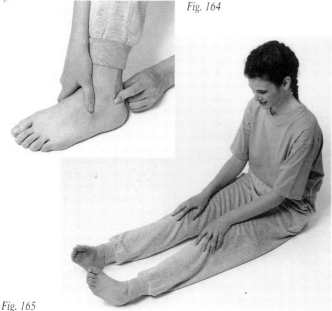

Fig. 164

Fig. 165

Feet

Bend your left leg once more and place your fingers underneath your left foot for support and your thumbs on top, just below your ankle bone. Your thumbs are now used to press along the meridian lines of your foot between your ankle and your toes. Pressure is applied in the spaces between the bones of your feet rather than on the bones themselves.

First, massage a line from your ankle down to the outside of the second toe. This is the line of the Stomach meridian (Fig. 166a & b). Keeping your fingers in contact with the sole of your foot, return your thumbs to just below your ankle but a little further over to the outside. Now massage a second line down to the outside of your third toe. In Japanese acupuncture this is known as the Stomach Branch meridian (Fig. 167a & b) which connects with the stomach and digestive system.

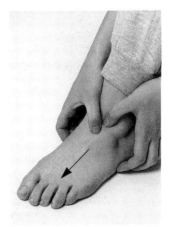
Fig. 166a

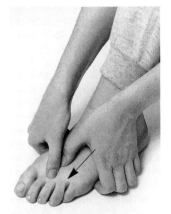
Fig. 166b

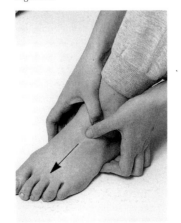
Fig. 167a

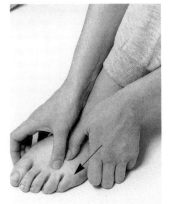
Fig. 167b

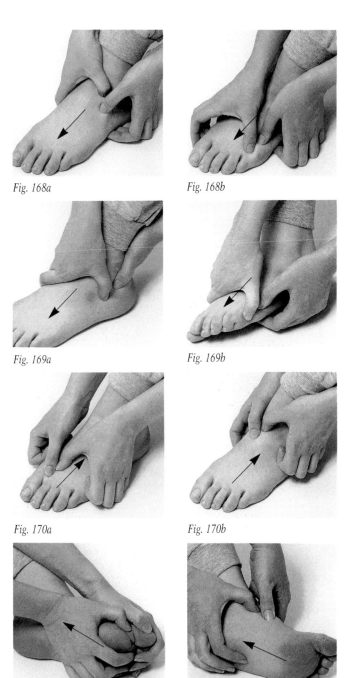

Fig. 168a

Fig. 168b

Fig. 169a

Fig. 169b

Fig. 170a

Fig. 170b

Fig. 171a

Fig. 171b

Again return your thumbs to just below your ankle bone, this time on the outside edge of your ankle. A line is now massaged down to the outside of your fourth toe. This is the line of the Gall Bladder meridian (Fig. 168a & b).

Now turn your foot in slightly, and return your thumbs to the outside of your ankle bone resting on the acupoint Urinary Bladder 60 (Fig. 169a). Massage with your thumbs down along the outside of your foot, following the line of the Urinary Bladder meridian down to the little toe (Fig. 169b).

Place your foot flat on the floor once more and press in with both thumbs on the inner edge of your big toe. Then work in a line up to your ankle bone. This is the line of the Liver meridian (Fig. 170a & b). Turn your foot sideways and place your thumbs on the outside of your big toe nail. Massage up along the inside edge of your foot to your ankle bone, following the line of the Spleen meridian (Fig. 171a & b).

Finally, turn your foot over and use both thumbs to press into the acupoint Kidney 1, located on your sole (Fig. 172a), and then to massage up the ankle following the line of the Kidney meridian (Fig. 172b).

Fig. 172a

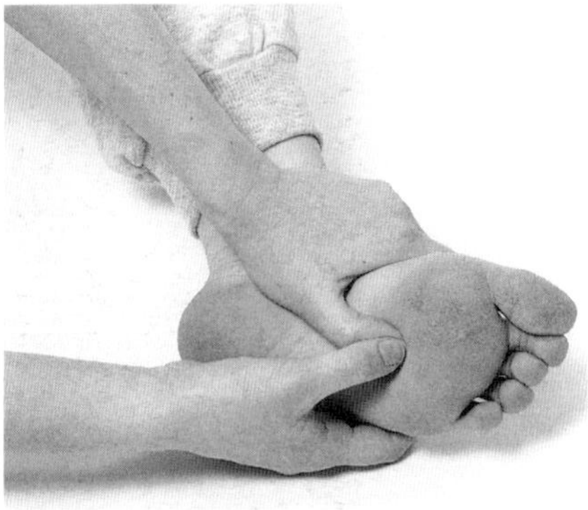

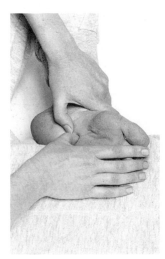

Acupoint Kidney 1

Location: In the depression underneath the ball of the foot, a third of the way along the sole.
Benefits: Eases sore throats, blurred vision and feverish sensations in the sole, and helps restore consciousness after fainting. A general tonic point to revive the spirit.

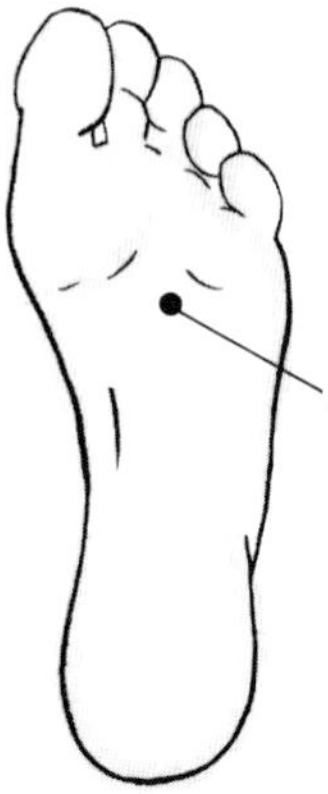

Acupoint: Kidney 1

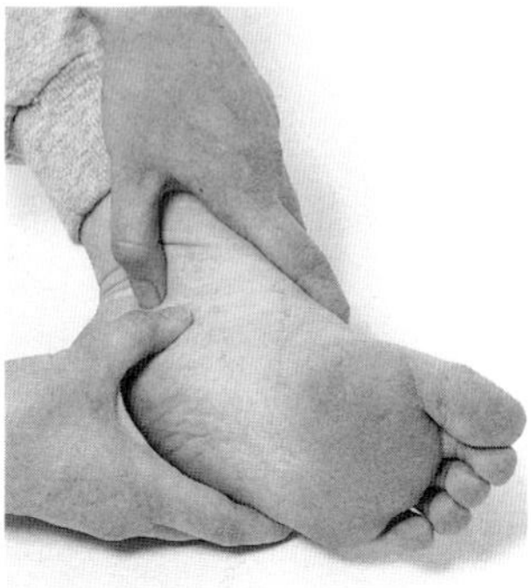

Fig. 172b

Massage of the acupoint Kidney 1 can also be done with your foot resting on your opposite thigh (Fig. 173).

Complete the foot massage by working all over your sole with both thumbs (Fig. 174). Apply touch-press-release with your thumbs, and support with your fingers.

For an invigorating effect, this can be repeated using a loose fist to

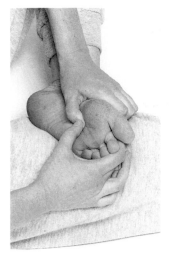

Fig. 173

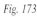

Fig. 174

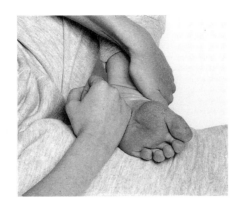

Fig. 175

pummel lightly (Fig. 175).

Throughout the massage, co-ordinate the movements with your breathing.

NOTE: If you wish to simplify the foot massage, instead of massaging each individual meridian line you can massage all across the top of the foot with the thumbs, working from the ankle down to the toes, and then up the side of the foot from the big toe to the inner ankle. Complete with the massage of the sole of the foot as before.

Benefits: Increases mobility of your foot and ankle and stimulates all the leg meridians.

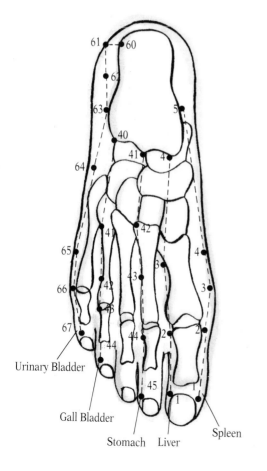

The meridians of the foot

Toes

Massage of your toes can be done with your leg bent or with your foot resting on your thigh.

Place your thumbs on top of your little toe and your index or middle fingers underneath, or vice versa if the foot is upturned on your thigh (Fig. 176). Using small rotating movements, massage from the base of your toe to the nail tip (Fig. 177). Repeat for your next toe and then massage each toe finishing with your big toe (Fig. 178).

If you have your foot in the raised position on your opposite thigh, you can also rotate each toe by holding it between the thumb and forefinger of your right hand, supporting with your left hand and moving your toe in both clockwise and anti-clockwise directions (Fig. 179).

Benefits: This releases tension in your toes and stimulates the start and end points of the leg meridians.

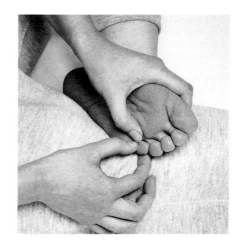

Fig. 176

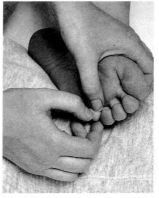

Fig. 177

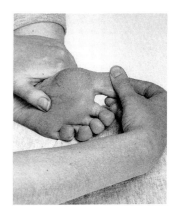

Fig. 178

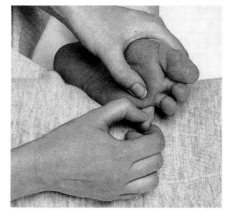

Fig. 179

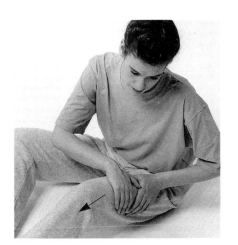

Fig. 180

Opposite Leg

Repeat the complete sequence for the right leg.

Completion

Stretch the legs out. Rub the palms of your hands together and then 'wash' **down** the **outside** of your left leg from the top of your thigh to your toes (Fig. 180), then **up** the **inside** of your leg to the groin (Fig. 181), and finally **down** the **back** of your leg to the heel and sole of your foot (Fig. 182). Repeat for your right leg.

This completes the massage of your legs and feet.

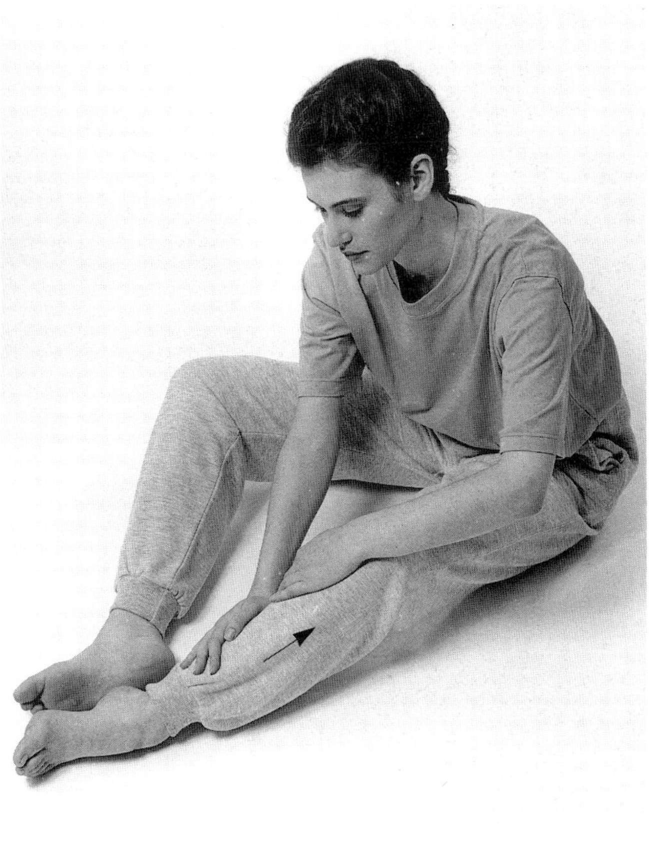

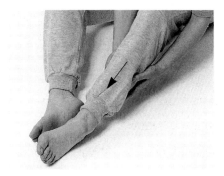

Fig. 181

Fig. 182

FINE POINTS

1 *Fine points of practice*

Amount of pressure

The pressure applied should always be firm but never uncomfortable or painful. By touching first (for example in the touch-press-release movements), you can always be sure that you are in the correct location before applying pressure. For example, when working along the ribs or feet, you can check that you are in the fleshy spaces between the bones so that pressure can correctly be applied there rather than on the bones themselves.

When using your fingers or thumbs, never apply force as this will leave them aching after the massage is finished. Instead check that after each application of pressure they are momentarily relaxed. By keeping your hands relaxed and the movements light, and by gradually building up the length of time you practise, your hands will become strong and it will be possible to apply firm pressure for sustained periods of time without any discomfort.

When applying pressure with your elbows, the amount of pressure can be controlled by the extent to which you lean your weight on to your elbow. Again, the pressure should be firm but comfortable.

Do not be afraid to press quite deeply into fleshy areas; for example, the abdomen. Here, you will find it is possible to press in at least an inch without any discomfort and you will experience a pleasant sensation of relaxation when the pressure is released.

When massaging acupoints, take care to apply the pressure vertically down into the point itself, or orientated slightly in the direction of flow of the meridian. If massaging acupoints along a limb, use a series of touch-press-release movements, or a number of small circular rotations, into the points. This helps to stimulate the flow of vital energy within the meridians.

Order and direction of massage

If you are doing the complete body self-massage, it is generally preferred to massage from your head to your toes. However, when massaging your arms or legs, do remember to work in the direction of flow of the meridian lines: i.e. **down** the **inside** of your arms and **up** the **outside**; and **down** the **back** and **side** of your legs and **up** the **inside**.

When working on your arms or legs, as already stated, you can choose whether to do one complete limb and then the other or to massage both together part by part. If you do give a complete massage on one side and then the other, make sure to regularly alternate the side that you start with. For example, on some days begin with the left arm and leg, and on other days, the right. Similarly, if you choose to work by body part: i.e., doing the upper part of your left arm and then your right arm, then the lower part for both and so on, make sure that you vary which arm or leg you begin with.

Doing this helps to balance the flow of energy between the different sides of your body, as well as muscular function.

Building up practice

Begin by practising for just ten to fifteen minutes a day. This should enable you to go through one body section at a time until you have mastered it. Once you are confident, begin to put the sections together until you can complete a full body self-massage. In the beginning, this may take about half an hour, but with practice you will be able to finish it within 15 minutes without difficulty.

In the early stages of practice, it is helpful to keep a notebook to record how you feel before, during and after practice. At first your body may find it hard to release tension and

tiredness but you will gradually find yourself relaxing as soon as you start the massage. You should also find that the vitalizing effects of the massage start to last longer.

As your hands become stronger and more used to the massage movements, it will be possible to build up your practice until you can massage for as long as you want.

Body awareness

As you prepare yourself with relaxation and breathing for the complete self-massage take care to notice any areas of tension, discomfort or pain in your body, and pay particular attention to these when you do the massage. Gentle rotating movements around the site of pain are very helpful in releasing pain, and the palm-squeezing technique effectively releases muscle tension.

As you work through the body, you may well find certain tender spots; these are often acupoints located on the meridian lines, and they give an idea of the functioning of the meridian and corresponding internal organ. For example, if you are massaging along your collarbone and find tender spots just beneath it, on the outer sides of the chest, these points are the start of the Lung meridian. They are often tender to touch when a person is suffering from a cold or building up to one. Massage of these points will help to clear the cold quickly and to prevent further colds.

If areas of tenderness are discovered when massaging your ears or abdomen, these can be cross-referenced with the diagrams which show the corresponding internal organs according to the oriental medicine system. It is important to remember that tenderness does not necessarily mean a physical abnormality of the organ; it can simply indicate a temporary imbalance as a result of a number of things, such as diet, particular activities, or even environmental conditions.

Accurate diagnosis using these systems requires considerable training and practice. However, as a general indicator, the microsystems can be very helpful in terms of increasing self-awareness of body changes on a day-to-day basis. Use of these systems, together with a developing sense of touch, can help to build up a close understanding of the body. This can enable you to know when to take rest, when to exercise, when to alter your diet and when to seek medical advice.

2 Adapting your practice

The speed of massage and type of pressure determines the effect of the massage: light and vigorous movements have a stimulating effect; slow, deeper movements have a calming effect.

If you are just massaging a part of the body, for example spending a few minutes on neck and shoulder massage at work, then apply average speed and pressure. Tune in to your body and feel what it needs.

You may also find that you intuitively adjust your massage according to factors such as body cycles, the weather and diet.

Body cycles

Women tend to have increased skin sensitivity and tenderness at acupoints around the time of menstruation. They may also experience changes in sensitivity in line with the cycles of the moon. Self-massage can be adjusted to accommodate this by simply applying lighter pressure at times of increased sensitivity. More vigorous self-massage in the week prior to menstruation can help to alleviate or prevent menstrual discomfort.

Weather

Some people are affected by the weather. The increase of electrical energy in the atmosphere before, or during, a storm can have a very disturbing effect. To alleviate this, slow rhythmical self-massage with deep pressure and plenty of the stroking movements to smooth down the body can help to release the build-up of energy and calm the affected person.

If you are particularly affected by cold and damp weather you will find that regular, vigorous self-massage will help to keep your joints mobile, and will minimize sensations of pain and heaviness.

In warm, sunny weather, the flow of energy in the meridians is quite active, and only light pressure is required to have an invigorating effect on them.

Diet

It is best to allow at least an hour after eating before beginning self-massage. Regular practice will also help you to determine the effects of certain foods on the body. The point Stomach 36 below the knees (see page 85) is a powerful indicator of the state of one's digestion. For example, if you have eaten something that disagrees with you, or that you may be allergic to, then this point will feel very tender indeed. If, on the other hand, the digestion is very weak, then even with firm pressure almost nothing is felt on the point. Regular massage of this point on both legs, together with abdominal massage, will help to strengthen digestion.

The harmful effect of excess sweet foods can also be demonstrated with self-massage. Try eating a bar of chocolate, and then apply pressure along the Spleen or Gall Bladder meridians on the sides of your foot (see page 91). You will immediately notice the dramatic sensitivity and tenderness along these lines as the corresponding organs deal with the effect of the sugary food on the body. The same effects can also be detected with other sweet foods.

Once again, this demonstrates how the self-massage system can be used to help you tune in to your body and its state of health.

3 Common questions and experiences

I feel faint during practice.

You probably have a tendency to hold your breath while concentrating on the movements; this is a common problem. The remedy is simply to focus on your breath while doing the self-massage to ensure that you are breathing freely and deeply at all times. Regular practice of the breathing exercises (see page 107) can also be helpful.

My hands ache after practice.

You are obviously applying too much pressure with your hands. Do not force or strain; keep the movements light and gentle, and begin by practising for short periods only. Gradually build up the length of time for practice as your hands become stronger. Regular practice of the finger and hand exercises (see page 110) will also help.

I am not sure how much pressure to apply.

The amount of pressure should be similar to that required for kneading bread. It should be firm but not painful. The amount of pressure needs to be adjusted according to the part of the body being massaged; fleshy areas can take more pressure than bony ones. Let your body tell you the amount of pressure it requires. After massage, each body part should feel relaxed and invigorated.

After massaging my legs, they tingle and feel as if they have grown in size.

These sensations are quite normal and result from the increased flow of blood and vital energy in your legs brought about by the massage. The sensations may be particularly noticeable when you first start to massage, but after some time, once the circulation and flow of energy in your legs improves, they will become less marked.

After I finish the massage, one side of my body feels different from the other.

This effect occurs because of energetic and muscular imbalances in your body. We have a tendency to predominantly use one side of the body for many habitual actions. For example, always sleeping on the same side of the body or always crossing the legs or arms in one direction. This creates patterns in your body structure which normally go unnoticed, as they are slowly built up over a long period of time.

One of the aims of self-massage is to regulate the circulation and flow of energy in your body as a whole. It takes a while to do this, and in the early stages the differences that already exist between the sides of your body become more apparent.

If the difference is very noticeable, then, when massaging your arms and legs, always begin by massaging on the stronger side of your body, followed by your weaker side. This will help to gradually build up your weaker side until the two are in balance.

After some time the differences will lessen and you will start to feel more balanced.

Do the meridians and acupoints actually exist?

Accounts of the meridians appear in ancient oriental texts dating back thousands of years. In the last 20 years there has been intensive scientific research to try to verify the existence of the meridians. Certain studies have suggested that the meridians are located in the connective tissue of the skin and that they appear to carry electrical current through the body. Experiments on specific acupoints have determined their location very precisely and also the effects of their stimulation, for example by acupuncture needles. To learn more about the meridians and the acupuncture system, see the 'Further reading' list at the end of this book.

I have difficulty locating the acupoints.

Locating acupoints does take a bit of practice. First, use the diagrams to get the correct position of the acupoint. Then apply light pressure using your most sensitive fingertip. When the point is located correctly, the fingertip will feel a small depression below the skin and there will be slight sensitivity in your body on the point itself. Occasionally, a tingling sensation may be produced or a 'running' sensation leading from the point along the body. This sensation is due to stimulation of the meridian line and is felt in certain sensitive people.

Another thing to remember is that the position of the acupoints can vary slightly from day to day. For example, the point Stomach 36 on the lower leg is quite active, constantly moving its position slightly. It is therefore best to develop sensitivity in the fingertips to locate the points accurately.

Can I do self-massage when I'm pregnant?

In the early stages of pregnancy there is no harm in doing self-massage, and indeed it may help to relieve aching or tension. However, do not apply pressure on the Spleen meridian points on the inside edge of your foot or the inside of your lower leg (see pages 87 and 91), as these are contraindicated during pregnancy. Simply apply light, stroking movements on these areas.

Gentle self-massage can be continued into the later stages of pregnancy if you are experienced in its practice and it feels comfortable. However, do not begin practice at this stage, but wait until after the birth.

4 Breathing exercises

Breathing is very important for the success of your massage. Try to make sure that at all times your chest is open, back straight and breathing is full and relaxed. It is helpful to spend a few minutes practising deep breathing before beginning self-massage. Some useful exercises are described below:

Awareness breathing

Either sitting in a chair or lying on the floor, close your eyes and focus on your breathing. Notice if you are using all of your chest, or only the upper, middle or lower part. Check to see if your breathing is quick or slow, shallow or deep, and whether the in- and out-breaths are of equal length.

By observing your breathing pattern, you will notice that when you are tired, worried or upset your breathing tends to become constrained and shallow, whereas when you are relaxed and happy, the breaths are fuller and deeper.

Regulating your breathing can help to increase the amount of energy in the body and to balance emotions.

Expanding breath

To regulate and expand your breath, start to apply a count to your breathing; breathe in to a count of four, and then out to a count of four; breathe in through the nose and out through the mouth. Do this for a minute and then change the count so that the exhalation is longer than the inhalation; for example, breathe in to a count of four, and out to a count of six or eight, whichever is most comfortable. Do not try to force or strain in any way, but find a count that will fit comfortably to your breathing. Spend several minutes breathing in this way and notice the relaxing effect it has on your body.

A prolonged, full out-breath helps to relax the body and calm the mind.

Diaphragmatic breathing

If you have a tendency to breathe shallowly at the top of your chest, it can be helpful to practise diaphragmatic breathing (Fig. 183). To do this, lie flat on the floor with your hands placed

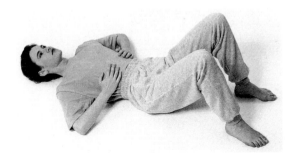

Fig. 183

over the lower ribs. As you breathe in, gently try to expand your lower abdomen so that your hands are raised upwards and outwards; as you breathe out, a light pressure can be exerted from your hands to press inwards and help expel any remaining air. Once again, try to make the exhalation longer than the inhalation.

This exercise can also be performed standing up with your hands resting on the sides of your rib-cage. Once again, as you breathe in, try to expand your ribs so that your hands are moved outwards. As you exhale, press in lightly with your hands to help expel any remaining air (Fig. 184).

Practising diaphragmatic breathing for a few minutes every day will dramatically change your natural breathing habits for the better!

Applying breathing to the massage techniques

When first learning the self-massage, it is best to simply try to maintain relaxed and full breathing throughout each movement. However, once you feel confident of the techniques, you can then apply the appropriate breathing to each one.

If you are slowly massaging a single point, then the general principle is to breathe out as

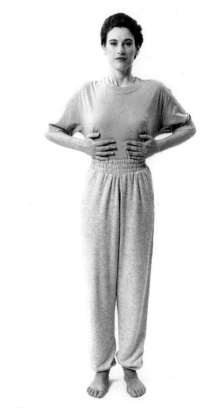

Fig. 184

you apply pressure, and to breathe in as pressure is released.

For example, in the eye massage where the touch-press-release movement is used, breathe in as you touch your thumb and finger to the bony socket under your eyebrow, and breathe out as you apply pressure. Then breathe in as you release the pressure and move your finger and thumb along to the next point. Breathe out as pressure is again applied and so on.

This helps to make the whole movement a very relaxed and flowing one.

If you find it takes too long to apply individual breathing for each technique, then apply rhythmical breathing according to the part of the body being massaged. For example, with the eyes you could breathe in as you massage up to the middle of your eyebrow, and breathe out as you massage down to the outer edge of your eye; and similarly, breathe in as you move to the centre of the bony socket below your eye and breathe out as you move on back up to the bridge of your nose. In this way, the breathing becomes rhythmical and in time with the movement.

If you are applying elbow pressure, then again you breathe out as weight is leaned on to the elbow and pressure applied, and you breathe in as the pressure is released.

With the palm-squeezing technique, the approach is slightly different: here you breathe in as you squeeze between your fingers and the heel of your palm, and then breathe out as you release. This is because we are working with a large area, rather than a single point, and the aim is to release tension in large muscles, for example at the back of the neck and shoulders. Breathing out as you release

the grip helps to release this tension.

When doing the stroking techniques, for example up and down your arms and legs, breathe in as you come up, and out as you go down.

For the abdominal rotation, breathe out as you press in with your fingers and in as you press in with the heel of your palm. In this way your breathing fits the undulating movement of your hands.

Breathing that is synchronized with the massage movements is said to facilitate the collection and distribution of vital energy in the acupoints and acupuncture meridians. With regular practice, your hands will become very sensitive and able to detect delicate changes in the flow of energy in the body. Different people experience this in different ways. For some it is a sensation in their fingers, for others a sensation in the palms of their hands.

Once this sensitivity develops, you will instinctively know where to apply pressure, for how long, and how deeply, and you will feel its effects. The only way to achieve this sensitivity is by regular practice, but it is surprising how quickly the skill can develop.

5 Finger and hand exercises

To strengthen your hands for self-massage it is advisable to regularly practise hand and finger exercises. It is also a good idea to incorporate such exercises into your 'warm-up' before beginning each massage. A sequence of hand and finger exercises is given below. Practise the whole sequence, or select some of the exercises each time you do a self-massage.

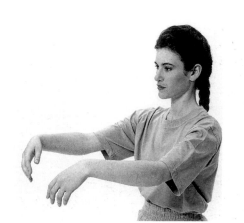

Fig. 185

Fig. 186

1 Stretch your arms out in front of you and shake your wrists loosely. (Fig. 185).

2 Bend your elbows, resting your hands on your shoulders as you breathe in (Fig. 186). Then, exhaling, stretch your arms out in front of you (Fig. 187). Repeat this movement five times. Then repeat a further five times but stretching your arms out to the sides (Fig. 188). Finally, repeat five times raising your arms above your head (Fig. 189).

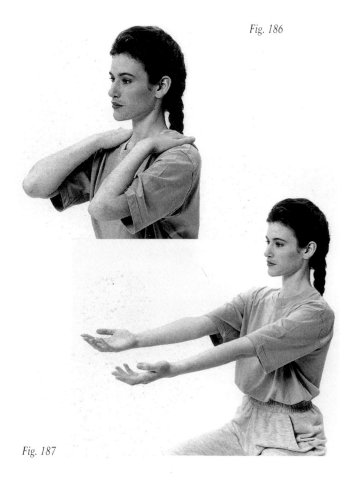

Fig. 187

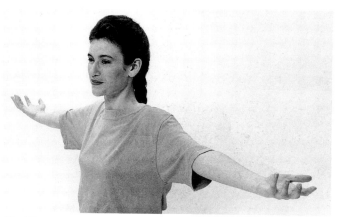

Fig. 188

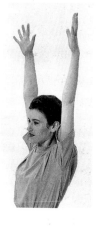

Fig. 189

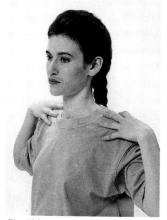

Fig. 190

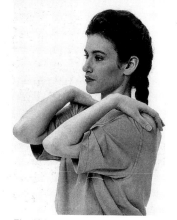

Fig. 191

3 Rest your hands on your shoulders with your elbows out to the sides (Fig. 190). As you inhale, draw your elbows up in front of your face (Fig. 191) and above your head (Fig. 192). As you exhale, lower them back down in a circular movement. Make five rotations in this direction and then five in the opposite direction, keeping the hands on the shoulders throughout. This exercise helps to release tension in the shoulders and increases circulation and the flow of energy down to your hands.

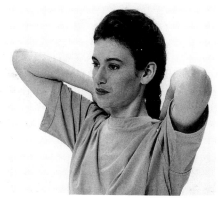

Fig. 192

4 Bending at the wrists, point the fingers down towards the floor then raise them to point towards the ceiling. Repeat this movement five times, breathing out as you point the fingers down, and in as you point them upwards (Figs. 193 and 194).

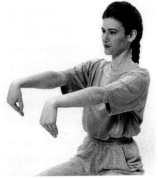

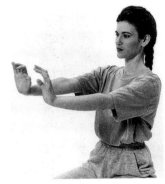

Fig. 193

Fig. 194

5 Stretch your arms out in front of you and make loose fists with your hands. Rotate your fists five times in one direction and five times in the other (Fig. 195).

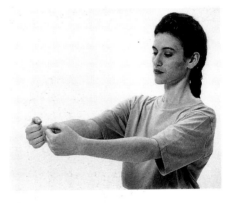

Fig. 195

6 Take your left hand in your right with your fingers around your palm and your thumb on the back of your hand. Gently press with your right thumb and stretch your left hand round, twisting at the wrist. Release and repeat, applying gentle pressure five times (Fig. 196). Then do the same for your right hand.

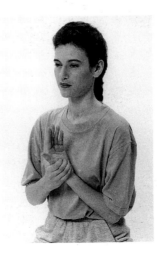

Fig. 196

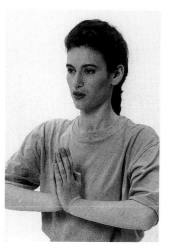

Fig. 197

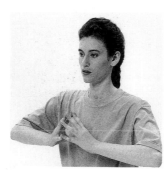

Fig. 198

7 Put your palms together, with the fingers touching but spread apart slightly (Fig. 197). As you breathe out, press your palms and fingers against one another; as you breathe in, relax them, but keep them touching. Repeat five times, then repeat the movement but with the palms apart and only your fingers touching (Fig. 198).

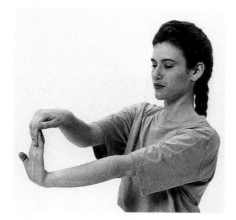

Fig. 199

8 Stretch your left arm out in front of you, place your right fingers over the top of your left hand and gently pull your fingers backwards. Release and repeat five times, then repeat for the right hand. Breathe out as you stretch back, and breathe in as you release (Fig. 199).

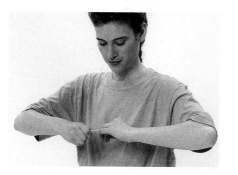

Fig. 200

9 Massage each individual finger, starting with your left hand (Fig. 200). Place your little finger between the thumb and fore-finger of your right hand and then use these fingers to massage from the base to the fingertip,

pulling apart with each hand as you do so. Repeat for each finger in turn and then do the same for the right hand.

10 Rest your little fingers lightly on a flat surface, such as a table or desk, or else on your thighs and lower your hands to stretch the fingers. Repeat for each of the other fingers in turn (Fig. 201).

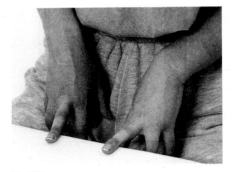

Fig. 201

11 To finish, rub the palms of your hands together and then shake your wrists out loosely once more.

If there is not time to perform all of these exercises, just select one or two that you find particularly helpful.

6 Massaging others

Once you have mastered the self-massage techniques, you can also show others how to perform them, or you can adapt them for use in massaging others. One way to do this is to give a massage of each of the acupoints shown in this book. Remember to massage the points on both sides of the body.

Alternatively, you could perform a relaxing massage of the feet or hands applying the same techniques as you used on yourself. For the hands, just sit opposite the person, and take their hand in yours. First use the stroking and palm-squeezing movements down the inside of the arm and up the outside of the arm several times. Then use the thumbs to work around the wrist, applying pressure on the acupoints as shown previously. Next press around the palms and then work down each finger.

To finish, repeat the stroking movements along the arm. Then change your position and repeat the procedure on the other arm.

Experiment with adapting each of the massage movements in this way.

APPENDICES:

KNOW YOUR BODY

1 *The skeletal system*

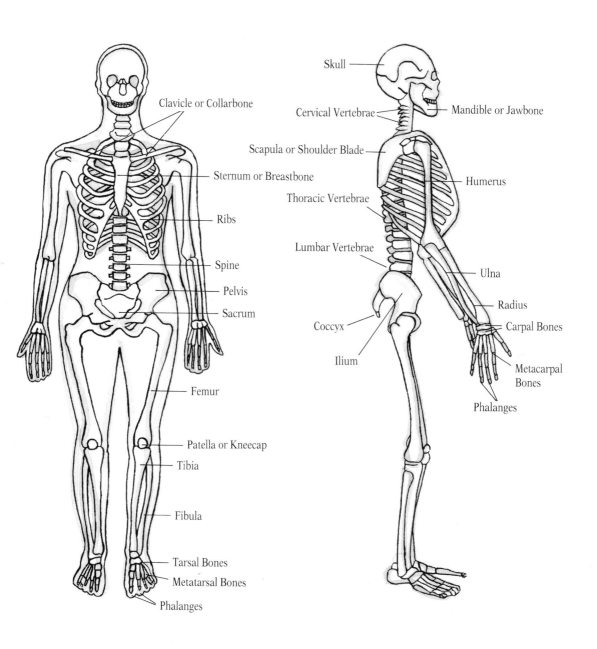

Clavicle or Collarbone

Sternum or Breastbone

Ribs

Spine

Pelvis

Sacrum

Femur

Patella or Kneecap

Tibia

Fibula

Tarsal Bones

Metatarsal Bones

Phalanges

Skull

Cervical Vertebrae

Mandible or Jawbone

Scapula or Shoulder Blade

Thoracic Vertebrae

Humerus

Lumbar Vertebrae

Ulna

Radius

Coccyx

Carpal Bones

Ilium

Metacarpal Bones

Phalanges

2 The muscular system

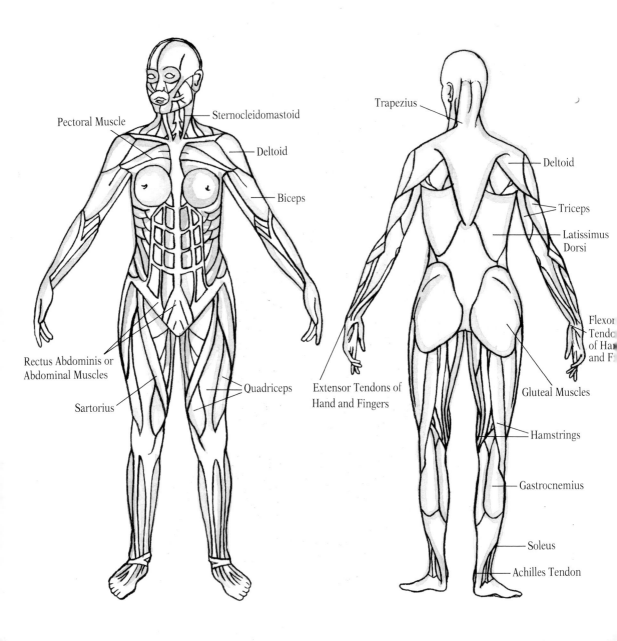

Pectoral Muscle

Sternocleidomastoid

Deltoid

Biceps

Rectus Abdominis or
Abdominal Muscles

Sartorius

Quadriceps

Extensor Tendons of
Hand and Fingers

Trapezius

Deltoid

Triceps

Latissimus
Dorsi

Flexor
Tendo
of Ha
and F

Gluteal Muscles

Hamstrings

Gastrocnemius

Soleus

Achilles Tendon

3 The vital organs

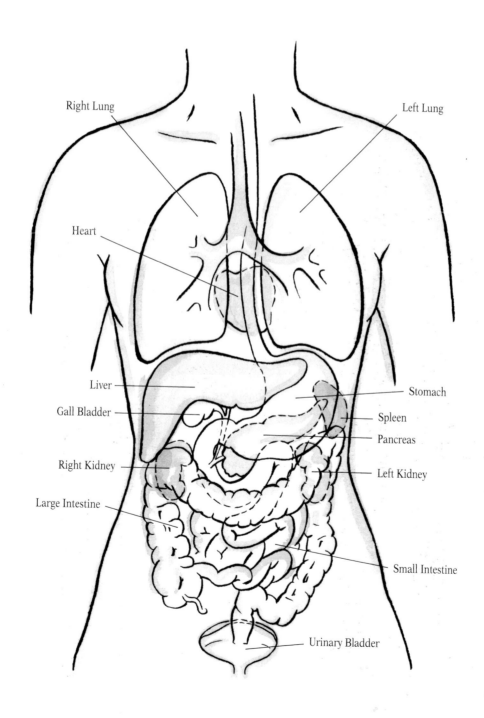

Right Lung

Left Lung

Heart

Liver

Gall Bladder

Stomach

Spleen

Pancreas

Right Kidney

Left Kidney

Large Intestine

Small Intestine

Urinary Bladder

4 The meridian system

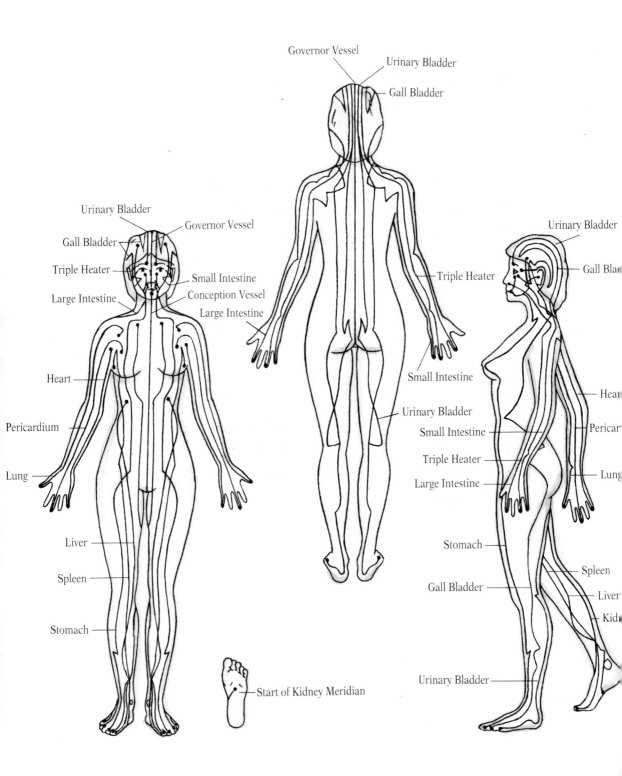

Governor Vessel

Urinary Bladder

Gall Bladder

Urinary Bladder

Gall Bladder

Governor Vessel

Triple Heater

Small Intestine

Large Intestine

Conception Vessel

Large Intestine

Heart

Pericardium

Lung

Liver

Spleen

Stomach

Triple Heater

Small Intestine

Urinary Bladder

Small Intestine

Triple Heater

Large Intestine

Stomach

Gall Bladder

Urinary Bladder

Urinary Bladder

Gall Bla

Hear

Pericar

Lung

Spleen

Liver

Kid

Start of Kidney Meridian

5 *Acupoint guide*

This section contains a handy alphabetical reference guide
to each of the acupoints used in the Self-Massage system
Folios in bold type show where illustrations occur.

Further reading

MASSAGE AND SHIATSU

Dawes, Nigel, & Harrold, Fiona, *Massage Cures: The Family Guide to Curing Common Ailments with Simple Massage Techniques* (Thorsons, London, UK, 1990).

Manaka, Dr Y., & Urquhart, Dr I. A., *Chinese Massage: Pain Control and First Aid* (Shufunotomo Co., Tokyo, Japan, 1984).

Masunaga, Shizuto, with Ohashi, Wataru, *Zen Shiatsu: How to Harmonise Yin and Yang for Better Health* (Japan Publications, Tokyo, Japan, 1977).

Ohashi, Wataru, *Do-it-yourself Shiatsu* (Unwin, London, UK, 1979).

ACUPRESSURE

Bahr, Frank, *The Acupressure Health Book: A Guide to Treatment for Pain and Illness* (Unwin Paperbacks, London, UK, 1982).

Jarmey, Chris and Tindall, John, *Acupressure for Common Ailments* (Gaia Books, London, UK, 1991).

ACUPUNCTURE AND THE MERIDIANS

Firebrace, Peter, & Hill, Sandra, *A Guide to Acupuncture* (Hamlyn, London, UK, 1988).

Kenyon, Dr J. N., *Modern Techniques of Acupuncture Vols. I, II and II* (Thorsons, Wellingborough, UK, 1983, 1983 and 1985).

Manaka, Dr Y., & Urquhart, Dr I. A., *The Layman's Guide to Acupunture* (Weatherhill, NY, USA, 1972).

Motoyama, Hiroshi, 'Functions of Ki and Psi Energy' in *IARP Journal* (Tokyo, Japan, 1981). (Available from Inokashira 4-11-7, Mitaka-shi, Tokyo 181, Japan.)

HARA

Durckheim, Karlfried Graf von, *Hara, the Vital Centre of Man* (George Allen and Unwin, London, UK, 1985).

Tohei, Koichi, *The Book of Ki: Coordinating Mind and Body in Daily Life* (Japan Publications, Tokyo, Japan, 1976).

ORIENTAL EXERCISES

Masunaga, Shizuto and Brown, Stephen, *Zen Imagery Exercises: Meridian Exercises for Wholesome Living* (Japan Publications, Tokyo, Japan, 1987).

Young, Jacqueline, *Vital Energy: Oriental Exercises for Health and Well Being* (Hodder and Stoughton, Sevenoaks, UK, 1990).

Footnote

The beneficial effects of this massage system are being researched. If you would like to contribute to this, please write to the address below giving details of your practice and the effects you have noticed.

Details of Self-Massage classes can be obtained from the same address. Please enclose a stamped addressed envelope with your enquiry.

Health Systems
PO Box 2211
Barnet
Hertfordshire
EN5 4QW
UK.

Index